LEAN ON ME

Hailey,

You need to experience rain in order to appreciate the sun!

LEAN ON ME

A STORY OF HOPE, HEALING AND HOLDING ON

SCOTT AND LINDA MALONEY

TATE PUBLISHING
AND **ENTERPRISES, LLC**

Published by Tate Publishing & Enterprises, LLC
127 E. Trade Center Terrace | Mustang, Oklahoma 73064 USA
1.888.361.9473 | www.tatepublishing.com

Tate Publishing is committed to excellence in the publishing industry. The company reflects the philosophy established by the founders, based on Psalm 68:11,
"The Lord gave the word and great was the company of those who published it."

Book design copyright © 2014 by Tate Publishing, LLC. All rights reserved.
Cover design by Junriel Boquecosa
Interior design by Caypeeline Casas

Published in the United States of America

ISBN: 978-1-63122-083-8
1. Biography & Autobiography / Personal Memoirs
2. Family & Relationships / General
14.04.14

CONTENTS

ACKNOWLEDGMENT

As my father has spent his career in aviation, I've often heard the phrase "take a look at things from 20,000 feet." He uses this phrase both literally and figuratively. That's what I tried to do while drafting this acknowledgment. There are so many to thank, I could fill a book. To the medical professionals at UMass Medical that saved my life, words alone cannot convey my gratitude. For the support of all those in my hometown of Plainville, MA and for the Becker College community, thank you. To my friends and relatives from near and far, your compassion was truly unforgettable. But most importantly to my family for being everything I needed, exactly when I needed it; my voice, my strength and my salvation.

Scott

To all those that had my back, when I was busy having Scott's back, thank you. Please know that whatever you did, however large or small, it did not go unnoticed. I remember every word of encouragement, every hopeful comment, every prayer and every card and letter I received. I remember the pats on my back and the soft smiles. I couldn't have been there for Scott if all of you had not been there for me. Although you have probably never been formally thanked, please know that you were always appreciated. This is my heart-felt thank you. Your prayers and mine were answered.

Linda

FOREWORD

Linda

The memories will never leave us. Our lives, all of them have been forever changed, for better or for worse. It has been over nine years since tragedy struck. In these nine long years, we have learned some of life's most valuable lessons. Children grew up and parents grew old, but all with such a unity of spirit, an undying determination, and a powerful force that until Scott's accident lay dormant within our family.

We are writing this memoir now for many reasons. First, to put closure on a life-altering experience, knowing that we survived, that we made it. Secondly, to recall the events of this ordeal at a quieter time and in detail so as not to forget and always appreciate the value of life. Lastly, with the hopes that readers understand the overwhelming need for aggressive advocacy. When those we love the most are unable to speak for themselves, a strong and determined voice is often times their only lifeline.

I feel so strongly about espousing the role of advocacy, but I also feel mindful and reserved. I know firsthand the necessity of this approach, but I also know with all of my soul and all of my being that my son is here today because of forces far more powerful than the medical professionals he encountered or any individual's devotion to his recovery.

His life was not over and his purpose not yet fulfilled.

Scott

September 17, 2004, I was a new twenty-one-year-old, senior in college, getting back into the swing of things. I had just moved back to Worcester, MA for my last year at Becker College. A big enough city despite being in Boston's shadow. Home of many colleges, college apartments, college bars, and college students. I was the second oldest of five children with two parents and one grandmother all under the same roof. How do I begin to describe several years of my life following September 17, 2004? Unimaginable grief, disappointment, and frustration, but at the same time, gratitude and appreciation overwhelm me as well. This accident tore my life apart, but through my recovery, in some ways, I feel that I am better than before.

The song titles in this book might need to be explained. The songs titled for each chapter are descriptive of the chapters themselves. The reason for such is twofold. Music has always been a big part of my life as well as in my early recovery. This was an uplifting way to put the final touches on what I hope you will find an uplifting story.

THE WAY WE WERE
THE WAY IT WAS/MY WORLD

Linda

The end of summer was nearing. The days were long with just a hint of autumn in the air to keep the nights cool and comfortable. Business was great as a real estate attorney. The last two years had been unprecedented. There was as much work as a small law firm could handle. My family life...as good as it gets. We all know that life is not perfect, people are not perfect, but if perfect was possible, I had perfect. Five incredible children and a best friend, Mike, whom I had the good sense to marry over a quarter of a century ago.

My oldest son, Michael, was in his second year of law school. At age twenty-four, he had already traveled much of the globe and was continuing to do so every chance he got. Winter break, spring break, and long weekends were cause for a quick trip to Europe, Asia, or anywhere that sounded remotely interesting. My children were all gifted, all with qualities that others admired. Michael's biggest attribute was his drive and determination, nothing was impossible.

Scott, age twenty-one, was always the life of the party. The one with the quick wit, the ridiculous retort, the one who could make you smile when you wanted to scream. He had a deep love of family that he wore like a badge of honor.

Jen, my only daughter and three years younger than her brother Scott, is strong and beautiful. She grew up surrounded by males, and as such, she learned how to be feminine, but with an inner strength that is unparalleled. She has that quiet assurance. She sees what needs to be done and does it, doesn't talk about it, just does it. I think she gets that from my mother.

Jason was sixteen. He was my baby for many years until the last of my babies was born. Strong and athletic just as his siblings before him, but Jason had a serious side. He was the worrier in our family. The one who would bring everyone back to reality when we would all fly off in different directions. Scott teased him with the nickname "Fedex," a term he picked up from the movie *Cheaper by the Dozen*, conveying the notion that he was dropped off at the doorstep and unlike the rest of us, serious and focused.

The last of the clan was Kyle, nine years Jason's junior and the spark that keeps the whole family on their toes. He is extremely bright and eager to constantly learn new things as is often the case for the youngest child. He is fortunate, he seemed to get a piece of the best in all of us. The sky is the limit for Kyle!

September arrived, and with it came a new adventure for us. We bought a log cabin home a few miles away from Sugarloaf in Carrabassett Valley, Maine. We decided we needed to have a family ski vacation home. It didn't matter that we couldn't ski well, and in fact, the family had only been skiing once before. (Where was Jason when we needed him?) This was a good thing. We were excited and couldn't wait to tell everyone. The school year was off to a good start, Jen was beginning her first year at a small private college in Worcester, just an hour or so from home. Scott ready to start his senior year at a neighboring college a few miles away from Jen. I was comforted to know that Scott was not far from her, so he could check in on her or just stop by to annoy her as all good brothers should do.

This year was not what I had imagined. This year would change our lives forever.

AND THE WAY IT WAS IN MINE

Scott

As I walked to my dorm after class, I pulled my cell phone from my cargo pocket and dialed. Jill's number was so embedded in my memory that I could type in the digits while barely glancing at my phone. As I waited for her to pick up, I shifted my green backpack in order to lighten the heavy load of books. Jill and I had our first major argument the weekend before, and remembering it brought up an angry feeling in the pit of my stomach. Even though we were over the fight, it still was a sensitive issue for both of us.

The voicemail picked up and I left a generic message asking her to call me back when she had a minute. There wasn't any immediate reason for me to talk to her, I just wanted to hear the sound of her voice and have her say something to make me smile, make me remember why I loved her so much. We had only been dating for a year and a month, but it seemed like a lifetime.

I fumbled with my keys while trying to get my fob that opened my dorm's door. Finally, getting inside, I took the sharp left to the stairs and climbed to the third floor. While juggling a water bottle and a cell phone in one hand and my backpack on one shoulder, I dropped my keys on the floor. "Crap!" I said out loud as I squatted down to pick them up. This was one more annoyance to add to an already long day. Work was starting to get on my nerves. I felt like a robot, given that it was a pretty repetitive job. I thought to myself I must say the phrase, "Expert Satellite, this is Scott..." over the phone about 1,800 times a day. I shouldn't complain though, the job was ideal for someone in my situation, a group of young guys right in the city with a less than stringent dress code. Working for a call center, I never had face-to-face contact with the customers, only talked to them on the phone. It could get tedious though, answering the same twenty questions.

I finally entered my room and took my shoes off immediately while placing my backpack in its usual corner in the walk-in closet. I then walked to my desk and sat down in front of my flat-panel computer monitor (it saves precious real estate on a dorm room desk) and proceeded to check my instant messenger (IM). I IM'd Jill again as an echo of the voicemail I left minutes before. I turned on some tunes on my computer's playlist and began my relaxation ritual for Thursday afternoons after class and before my company's first softball game.

My friend Pete was coming up the following night; he was originally set to come up that night, but the softball game had postponed those plans. As I took a light mid-afternoon snooze, I fell asleep with thoughts of my girl-friend, Jill, dancing through my head. I was living alone, I was a good student (by my subjective standards), I had my family within an hour of school, I had a girlfriend who was crazy about me as I was for her, and an array of friends around me. Could life be any better?

Crap! How could I have not set an alarm? How could I have slept through four of Jill's calls? How could I have overslept? Well, the bright side was that those at work wouldn't be too disappointed, how could they be? I was missing a softball game, not a workday. I quickly slugged some lemonade, knowing exactly where my ball glove was, as well as the cleats, ball playing pants, and the shirt I was going to wear. All on top of my "big three," which were my (1) wallet, (2) keys, and (3) cell phone. I knew never to go anywhere without those three things because there wasn't a situation in the world where it wouldn't be handy to have one of them. One of the benefits to being a neat freak was that no matter how late you were going to be, you always knew where to find things.

I quickly got changed and decided that I'd call Jill on the way to the game. Besides, now that I thought about it, we were just playing some investment company from one of the Worcester suburbs, a walkover of a team, a bunch of middle-aged men who wanted to play against some twenty-somethings to try to stand up to Team Expert Satellite. We were unstoppable, I was unstoppable. Not a ball could get by me as catcher. Just like the many balls life had thrown at me: school, working a full-time job, a full-time girlfriend, friends, and an extremely full-time family. You couldn't say we had ringers because they honestly worked as employees at Expert Satellite, but they just happened to be members of the Worcester State College baseball team. Being the natural athlete I was I fit right in with these guys. By the time I got there, it was already the bottom of the fourth and it was only a seven-inning game. We were on top of the competition 9-1, so it was kind of trivial to send me in. But I still managed to get a couple of at bats. The highlight of my three innings was making it to third on a bunt. I hit a bunt to drive in the only runner from third base. The base runner got in a pickle, but was eventually able to make it home. Meanwhile, I was trying for second, the catcher overthrew it, which allowed me to make it to third while standing up. Just an example of how "things work out." This used to be a popular quote from my older brother, Michael. So we ended up as the victors, of course. My coworkers all went out for a few drinks, but I declined the invitation because I had other plans with a friend, my old roommate, Ben.

Ben was someone I grew very close to in my years at Becker College, and I felt that I was a better person for having known him. Bad roommates and different campuses, it seemed like our friendship was put to the test and it came through with flying colors. So I left the team driving back to the dorm in my 1996 Ford Probe. I took the scenic route through Elm Park, realizing that this was one of my first times returning to my dorm this year. *Soon enough*, I thought. "This'll be same ol', same ol." Turns out it would be one of my last as well.

Benji, as I affectionately came to call Ben, and I had a brisk walk that was only .7 miles from my dorm to Leitrum's, a local college bar that was the place to see and be seen throughout Worcester. The night was cool but not too cool. The stars were in line for this to be an unforgettable weekend.

Pete, "Pistol Pete" as my father knows him, was a good friend of mine from home. It was easy to separate my worlds (borrowed from NBC's *Seinfeld*), college from hometown. He, along with most of my friends from home, were all a year younger than me. I'm not sure if it was because I was always the youngest in my class or was always the most immature in my class, either way hanging out with those one year younger and a class below me made for a good fit.

Pete and I had been friends since my sophomore year in high school, his freshmen (thus the concept), and we had been really good friends since what became known as "The Sleepover of 98." We were both pretty good wrestlers. One night, our high school wrestling team captain decided that because he lived only a few streets away from the school and we had to be at the school early the next morning for a tournament, he would have the whole team sleep over to save time.

Well, me being the hell-raiser I was, decided to pack everything for this sleepover and I mean everything; paint grenades, eggs, smoke grenades, firecrackers, rolls of toilet paper, the list goes on. I was like a Boy Scout "always pre-pared" for any situation, except I forgot the basic necessities of a sleepover, blanket and pillow. I still remember what my punch line was over fifteen years later, when asked "Why in God's name did you bring all of these munitions?" My reply was a question, "Which neighbors don't you like?" My witty remark got them to laugh, thus my objective was completed.

I, being the man I was back then, didn't bother to say I slipped up and forgot a sleeping bag and pillow, so as the night wore on, I made a plan. I saw this short, husky body with this enormous blanket, and he even had a pillow that looked as though it could fit a spare head or two. As night turned to early morning, the feet that separated the two of us diminished to inches; it was only a matter of time before we were embracing, er, I mean, "hugging" each other. Pete was the first one awake the next morning when I heard the shrill scream deafen my left ear and wake up the room, nay, the house. It was only a matter of time before we laughed about the situation, and now, it's part of the folklore as to why my high school's wrestling team had such a tightly knit bond of friendship.

So after a quick nap on Friday afternoon, I took a shower on the second floor, because the third floor only consisted of my room and one other dorm room, that was it. The room across from mine was large and designed to fit four freshman guys; one of them played guitar, another played mandolin and guitar, and the other two played soccer. A little bit younger, but my type of people. I, too, had played soccer my first two years of college before switching over to Cross-Country in its inaugural season, my junior year. I played guitar, sang (#debatable), and played harmonica. I could even beat my way through a set of drums if necessary. I played with two friends from home who were pretty serious musicians. Pete, Mike, and Scott were our names so logically we chose the name of our band as PMS.

I couldn't or shouldn't have stayed out so late because I had work the next morning. But I just didn't like the idea of work interfering with college life. But you need to make college money to buy college beer, right?

So the night came; right after I napped, I had two hot dogs and a starving man's portion of fries on the side. The dining hall was an easy commute, the next building over from my dorm.

Soon, Pete was there and scoping out my new dorm and the plethora of "Alpha Sierra Alpha Foxtrots" (Available Single Attractive Females). Pete hadn't been in my room for more than a few seconds and he already had a guitar in his hands.

I introduced him to my neighbors. He only seemed mildly interested, but when I explained to him that they played instruments too, he became wildly interested. Tonight was going to be just fine. The night was underway with Pete and I having one or two beers with the freshmen. Pete taught one of the freshmen some tricky scale on the guitar while he taught Pete the basics of mandolin. Soon we were off to an off-campus apartment for more partying.

We called it a night around the same time that Ben and I had on the previous night, around closing time for the bars, which in Massachusetts is 2:00 a.m. As Pete and I were walking back to my dorm we got a little lost/disoriented, possibly because it was so late, dark, and rainy, possibly, no, most likely because of the alcohol or because it was my first night on foot in a part of the city just a few blocks from my dorm, but these were unfamiliar blocks.

Eventually, we made it back to the dorm. The same freshmen, who we were jamming with us a few hours prior, were coming home from another party, just a few steps in front of us. They held the door open. We trudged our way up three long flights of stairs and decided to stop by their room. One of them was juggling a soccer ball, maximizing the roominess of his quad, another was playing guitar and two came in right in front of us. So we obviously didn't go to bed, we went in and joined the Hendrix wannabe and showed him the riff we decided he was going for. I remember it very well but don't remember how to play it, ZZ Top's

"La Grange." That song has the ability to put you down when you are feeling wide awake if it's played right. With Pete there, you knew it would be played right.

Eventually, we wanted to call it a night, which we tried to; we went across the hall to my room and then I realized I had forgotten something.

My keys, my keys, *my keys*! How could I have forgotten one-third of the big three? I frantically searched my front pockets, back pockets, and cargo pockets with no luck! I still to this day can't believe I forgot one of the Big Three. How could my comedic OCD (obsessive compulsive disorder) fail me? I never went anywhere without my Big Three. They weren't at Paul's apartment, I know that much. Could they possibly be on my fridge in the SIDBTCA (Standard Issue Designated Big Three Containment Area) PMS always used military terms and acronyms instead of civilian terms, "standard issue" to replace "regular."

I checked my cell phone for the time, 2:19 a.m. "Crap!" I said aloud, that was too late for campus police to respond to a "locked out" call without them thinking something shady was afoot. The police would surely know that forgetting keys was an understandable mistake that any college kid could make, but the fact that it was almost 2:30 a.m. would raise eyebrows, as to what I was doing up at this hour on a Friday night/Saturday morning. Alcohol? I hadn't bought any alcohol for the freshmen, but I still didn't want to be the one responsible for getting them busted. Just think, me a twenty-one-year-old senior, legal to drink, responsible for all these freshmen getting caught with alcohol. The student athletes who could get suspended from games or worse yet suspended for the season, not exactly the kind of thing a kid would like to explain to his parents over the phone.

So I made the simple uncomplicated decision to go out from my hallway window, across a small distance on the roof and into my dorm room window, nothing too drastic. Just your basic "MacGyver-esque" maneuver. I would show these freshmen the steps necessary to hide "dorm drinking."

So I climbed out the window. *Jeez*, I thought to myself. *It's really gotten rainy out.* There was what I thought a strategically placed tree branch that I could climb out on from the third-story hall window and from there I could climb in my dorm window. Just then, I felt the wet bark of the tree start to slip from my fingers.

I don't actually remember the fall. There is a vague recollection of paramedics telling me not to move. That was my last memory for a very long time.

KNOCKIN' ON HEAVEN'S DOOR

Linda

September 18, 2004, my perfect life stopped. At 3:00 a.m. on that morning, we received a phone call from Becker College. My son Scott had been hurt in a fall. The school told us that he was being transported to UMass Medical Center. We should meet him there. We immediately got dressed and headed out. Although late, both my husband and I had no idea of what the night would bring. You see, with five children, four of them boys and very sports-minded, we were used to regular trips to the ER, stitches, broken bones, etc. We could handle this. Before leaving, I woke my mother, who lives with us, to let her know we were leaving for the hospital, nothing to worry about, no need to wake the others...or so we thought.

Mike and I have been together so long. We dated as teenagers, married as young adults, and have been devoted best friends for as long as I can remember. Oftentimes, we were able to answer each other's questions before they were asked or know what each other was thinking. This phenomenon is shared by many a couple, or so I've been told.

As we drove toward the hospital on that rainy fall night, it happened again. We both felt it, at once, this visit to the ER was different. Panic set in.

When arriving at the hospital, we were immediately escorted into a small room by two young residents. The older of the two gave us the news we were not prepared to hear. Scott had taken a fall from two and a half stories and had taken the brunt of the fall to his head. We were told to say good-bye. We were told that Scott was gone, brain dead. We pleaded with the doctors to do something. They showed us CT scans on a computer screen next to his bed to illustrate the traumatic brain injury (TBI), the damage that had been done and insisting their was no hope. Here we stood surrounded by competent, caring, and compassionate professionals, while watching our son in disbelief.

In the midst of all this organized chaos of medical professionals doing what they do, of wires and tubes and the sounds of an ICU, there appeared a woman unlike the others that surrounded us. She was a small black woman with a thick island accent and although different than all the others, she was noticeably quite comfortable in her surroundings. I would later come to find out that her name was Mercy Essien, but not until two years later find out why Mercy was with us that evening.

Mercy quietly and unassumingly approached me. She asked if I would like her to pray for our son. I told her very directly and what I remember as being in a somewhat curt voice that my son was not going to die and I did not want prayers for his death, his soul. Grabbing my hand, she assured me that these prayers would be for his life, so his life might be spared. All the while I remember thinking, why are all these professionals with advanced medical degrees and so many years of specialized training allowing her to control the situation if only for a few critical minutes? I later came to realize it was because they felt their work was done, what was left was compassionately caring for Scott's family in our time of grief. And so it was she prayed, instructing me to hold her hand, place my other hand on Scott, and close my eyes. The words of the prayer I never quite recalled, only that it was short and sweet and to the point. During her prayer, I felt something I had never felt before in my life and only once since then. It was a surge of energy, of power so strong from her hand to mine to Scott. I opened my eyes quickly. I had to look at all the others in the room to see if they had witnessed this energy force. My husband on the opposite side of the bed and the many other nurses and doctors in this tiny room were not struck by what I had just felt. Mercy let go of my hand, turned to me, and repeated that she would pray for my son and then left as quietly and anonymously as she had entered. Again, we pleaded with the doctors to operate, to do anything to give him a chance. What if this were your son, we begged, later learning that the surgeon we were speaking to did have a son, just Scott's age.

At that moment, one of the residents attending to my son spoke out. I recall how he spoke to the neurosurgeon, Dr. McGillicuddy, Mike, and I. "I'm not sure, but I may have, I think I might have seen the slightest flicker in Scott's left eye. Again, I'm not sure." This was enough, just the slightest bit of hope, to allow Dr. McGillicuddy to operate, but not before explaining to us that our son had less than a two percent chance of even making it into the operating room, let alone through the surgery. We were told further that even if by some miracle he survived the surgery, he more than likely would never be the same again, never be able to think, walk, or talk again.

Our families were called. Our children arrived with my mother, Helen, and my sister Carol and her husband, Tom. They were allowed to see Scott, but only for seconds before the surgery. He was in a coma and on a ventilator. This was an unbearable sight for my children to see their strong, independent, and outgoing brother, teetering on the brink of death, but they had to see him. My oldest son Michael was not at home that night. We finally got hold of him at his cousin's in downtown Boston, but the doctors could not wait any longer. Scott needed to be prepped for surgery. We waited downstairs by the entrance to surgery to give Scott one last kiss and tell him, plead with him to hear us, and fight for his life. He needed to keep fighting. Just as they wheeled Scott into surgery, Michael arrived. This usually calm young man was out of control. At 6'2", two hundred pounds, and all muscle, he can be somewhat intimidating, especially when spewing words that we had never before heard from his mouth. A surgical nurse heard him, saw his pain, and with compassion and wisdom beyond her years, she took him aside, dressed him in surgical garb, and told him that he had seconds to go in and tell his brother he loved him and then let them do their jobs to try to save his life. I don't know who that woman was, I never got her name, but I will never forget her.

Surgery was to last about four hours. We arrived at the waiting room to find it overflowing with family and friends. It was barely 6:00 a.m., and there were more than a hundred people already there. They were piled in next to each other, chairs were set up in the hallway. Scott had touched so many lives in such a short time. Mike and I were speechless surrounded by all those we loved, waiting for the phone to ring in the waiting room, but praying that it wouldn't. I couldn't bear to hear the news.

At 9:00 a.m., we were informed that the surgery was successful, a piece of damaged tissue was removed from his temporal lobe, but luckily, Dr. McGillicuddy explained, that was the good news. The piece that needed to be removed was a portion of the brain that none of us use. As he explained, I kissed him, hanging on to every ounce of hope. He quickly dissuaded my enthusiasm and continued to explain that he removed all the blood they could, but that the rest was out of his hands, the next forty-eight hours would be critical. Scott's brain had been forced to one side in the fall, and they were not sure if it would move back to center as it should. Only time would tell. Further, there would be an issue with more swelling, and he went on to explain the treatments that would be used if swelling persisted. The treatments seemed to be as risky as the swelling itself. A craniotomy was performed (a portion of Scott's skull was removed) and placed in a deep freeze for months until they were sure all of the swelling had subsided.

Mike and I clung to each other, those days, weeks, and months to follow. Our lives stopped, our careers ceased, and our other four children became secondary to the needs of Scott. But that was okay, we could do this. We dealt with tough times before. I still recall the words of one of the physicians in those very early days of Scott's injury. "If your son survives, the process of recovery, to the extent one recovers, is a very trying time. It makes strong families stronger and weaker families fall apart." We were strong, we knew that, we had an undeniable family bond that could not be broken. Looking back, I've come to realize that there are no words to explain what was to lie ahead, perhaps that is best because enormous amounts of energy are needed just to cope with every hour of every day, and the challenges and decisions that must be made.

Mike and I slept next to Scott the night after the surgery. He was in ICU, in a single room, and they seemed to bend the rules. We held each other all night as we whispered to Scott continually telling him how much we loved him and how he needed to keep holding on. Keep fighting.

Twenty-four hours passed, then forty-eight. We kept praying. The bargains you make with God are amazing. Just let him live. We'll make him well. We will do whatever it takes, we will bring him home and make him Scott again.

As time passed, the crowds didn't dissipate, they grew. Both Mike and I have large extended families, and Scott had an amazing group of friends because, as we would come to learn during these long arduous hours, he was an amazing friend. The hospital staff soon realized that the crowd was too large for this particular waiting room and asked if we could have everyone move down the hall to a larger room in a more secluded area. These people waited, unable to visit Scott, but there to support us. They needed to be there, for themselves as well as for us.

Mike was a corporate pilot for an insurance company in western Massachusetts. He had been employed there for about fifteen years after his service in the Marines as a helicopter pilot. His flight department and the company as a whole showed overwhelming support. It is the support of so many friends, loved ones, and even complete strangers that got us through these times. During the first few weeks of Scott's hospital stay, we were compelled to make medical decisions, life and death decisions. We had to educate ourselves, ask the right questions, understand the answers, and deliberate, knowing all the while that time was of the essence and our son's future might well depend on our answers.

Fortunately, for all of us, Scott did not have shy, unassuming parents. For that matter, no one in the family is quiet or unassuming. We knew enough to speak up when needed, to listen when necessary, and to constantly ask questions. Everything needed to make sense to us before we would agree to the treatment. I've always believed that fate plays a big role in our lives, but so, too, does free will. It's tough to forecast where one begins and the other ends.

I began my college career at age thirty, much later than most. I was pregnant with my fourth child, Jason. I did so knowing that law school was my goal, but didn't mention that to anyone, not until I was well on my way through my undergrad program. I thought it would seem too far-fetched at the time for anyone to take me seriously, since I barely graduated high school. I went through high school during the Boston Bussing Crisis, left in my senior year, and ended up graduating, taking evening classes at an outlying high school. There were seven people in my graduating class (not much of a graduation). Although I always considered myself to be an intelligent person, there was a part of me that felt lessened because I had not continued my education. The short version of the story is I finished my undergrad, testing out of as many courses as possible, entered law school, and graduated from Massachusetts School of Law several years later. Who would have thought then that three of my children would follow in my footsteps? Beyond that, who would have thought that in my mind, at least, my law degree gave me the confidence I needed to fight the battles necessary during the darkest time in our lives. Mentally, I was stronger and more confident than before. I honestly believe that it was some of the obstacles I overcame while putting myself through law school, raising a family and working full-time that gave me the self-assurance I needed to fight alongside my husband, the toughest battle of our lives.

The intubation tube was replaced by a tracheal tube; it was expected that Scott would not be breathing on his own for a while, if ever. A feeding tube was placed in his stomach, and a monitor in his head to check for intracranial pressure. There was no time for sadness or depression. There would be time for that later. As the days passed and hope grew that Scott would survive, the hospital began to limit the amount of time we could spend in the room with him, so our days and nights were spent in the waiting room. We were allowed minutes out of every hour. The waiting room became our home. We also booked a hotel room across the street from the hospital so the kids could shower and change, but for the most part, across the street was too far away for Mike and I.

CRAZY

Linda

Our lack of sleep at times made us giddy and our behavior sometimes not exactly what it should have been. Mike and I both dealt with our pain differently. We were so united, but had to cope in our own way. Mike and Scott are the big history buffs in our family. As such, Mike decided that when Scott recovered, he was going to punish him for the hell that he put us through by caning him, much like they did years ago in Thailand. He would tell everyone this story and invite them to a big caning party at our house when this nightmare was over. His story was strange, his reasoning bizarre, but it was okay because he was relaying it to family and friends. They understood that this was Mike's way of intertwining humor and grief. If anyone would have understood, it was Scott. Scott is in many ways a clone of his father. His invites to such a party were okay, that is until he invited a social worker to the party. Per hospital policy, she came to speak with us and assess our situation. I kept explaining to her that it was merely a joke, a warped type of humor, but I'm not so sure she understood. She was young, new to her job, and probably had a story or two to tell about the Maloney family.

Some family members tried maybe a little too much to make our hospital waiting room feel like home. They brought in a coffeepot, some DVDs, and blankets. But when one of them suggested a microfridge, we all lost it, particularly Jason. He pulled me aside, held on to my arms so he could hold me at attention, and said, "Make them stop, this is not our home." I did. They listened.

It wasn't just our extended family that got carried away, we were all bordering on insanity. Luckily, it seemed to be at different days and times. That way the sane one in the group could take care of the others who had lost their way.

It was mid-morning on a Monday. I had gone down to the cafeteria for a cup of coffee. Upon returning, I met a woman who looked visibly upset leaving the waiting room. As she was alone and I felt blessed that throughout all of this nightmare I was never alone, I stopped to ask if something was wrong. How could I help? It seemed her son had been badly injured in an accident. I asked if she would come and sit for a while. She remarked that this particular waiting room was reserved for one family and she was heading down the hall to another. I didn't quite understand, I told her that it was my family in there and urged her to join us as there must be some misunderstanding. She politely, and without the slightest amount of bitterness in her tone, refused. She was too overwhelmed with her own nightmare to be disconcerted or offended by the crazies in that waiting area.

Before I was able to utter a word as to what happened during my ten-minute walk for coffee, Jason approached me. Apparently, my husband and my mother, the woman whose genuine goodness is unmatched, had told this woman that the waiting room was occupied. We were the crazies! I talked to Mike and my mom about what had happened, Mike insisted that this was our waiting area and my mother selfishly agreed. There wasn't a selfish bone in their bodies, but they were so blinded by their love and devotion to Scott, they could see nothing else. This argument would be better left for another time.

Those first few days in the ICU when Scott's risks were the greatest, he was fortunate to be under the care of a nurse we came to call Big Bob. He had rules about everything, when we could visit, who could visit, what to talk about when we visited, and so much more. At first, I was upset by all these rules; I felt that I needed to be there constantly. I not only needed to watch over Scott, but I needed to watch over Big Bob to make sure he was watching over Scott. But I soon came to realize that this large bearded man with glasses, who did not look the part at all, was probably one of the most nurturing, caring nurses I have ever met. His job was to take care of Scott, not Scott's family, and he was doing it well.

TO EVERYTHING THERE IS A SEASON

Linda

After about ten days in ICU, the staff began talking to us about moving Scott to a regular floor. This scared me tremendously. He was still unable to breathe, in a coma, and needed the constant round-the-clock care that ICU provided. We were able to delay the move a couple of days, but the hospital soon insisted he must be moved. He was no longer what they considered to be in need of critical care. Although we should have taken this as a time of rejoicing, perhaps he was getting better, we didn't. We knew it was too soon and were very uncomfortable with the level of care he would receive on a regular floor. There is just not enough staffing.

We realized then that our new life was not going to be over anytime soon. We had to rethink our plan. It was time to get the rest of the family's life in order. We had to move out of the waiting room and the hotel. Time for our children to get back to school. They could commute back and forth, but they needed a routine. Mike and I talked, we would both stay at the hospital during the day and one of us would stay each night, the other going home to be with the rest of the gang. I didn't have to worry about my little guy, never once. I have a mother that is like no one else. I never asked, never had to, I just knew that my mother would be what she always was, incredible. She did everything, took care of Kyle, homework, driving, laundry, and life in general and yet seemed to be at the hospital all the time. I missed my children terribly in all of this, but I never once worried about their care. I never had to because I have a mother that really is like no one else.

So it was the night before Scott's transfer to a regular floor, we packed up the waiting room, what had become our home away from home. Loading the cars up with whatever had been collected over the last couple of weeks was no small task. There to help us was Scott's good friend Michelle. She was someone who Scott had met in high school and theirs was a friendship that continued all through college. She was a year younger and was attending a neighboring college in Worcester. She was one of those friends among friends, spending hours upon hours just sitting, waiting, and praying. We learned things about Scott from Michelle and others that maybe we didn't need to know. But while he was there fighting for his life, his adventures and the crazy stories of college antics were exactly what we needed to hear.

Michelle also learned a few things about us (Mike and I), maybe things she didn't need to learn. One afternoon, after classes, Michelle came by to check on Scott and sit for hours, as she did so many days. She sat down and, with a quick hello, asked Mike how Scott was doing. Mike didn't answer. He couldn't because he was very busy playing solitaire (too busy to speak). He had played earlier in the day and won (if that's what you call it in solitaire). Immediately after winning, Scott showed signs of improvement. They were minimal, so minimal, in fact, that I don't remember exactly what occurred, but what I do remember is Mike's reactions. He insisted that he finish the game he was playing, winning again could mean more improvements for Scott. This went on for a few days. When your child's life is on the line, all semblance of reason is gone.

While loading things and transferring from one car to another, deciding who would be driving which cars, I felt it again. We were in the parking garage, second floor, of a four floor garage. My son, Michael, and I were crossing paths as we transferred items, when there it was, that "surge of energy," a kind of rush of air that encompassed only the two of us. Mike, Jen, Jason, and Michelle were there also, but this surge only hit the two of us. I looked at Michael, and before I uttered the words "Did you feel that," he responded "I did, I know." I took this as a sign, just like before, that we were being watched over, that somehow through all of this nightmare, God was with us. Michael and I stopped, only for a moment. We both smiled. Michael spoke with calm emotion and said, "He's going to make it, we're going to make it." For only the second time in my life, I knew it,

God, or whatever word or phrase you may use to embellish the notion of a higher power, was with us then, for that moment, just as he was that first night. He was watching over our family.

I needed to know that Scott was going to make it, that my family would someday be whole again. I needed a dose of faith so I could continue through this tunnel and find our lives on the other side. I got it!

I HOLD ON

Linda

Transfer to a regular floor meant no more one-on-one care. Now the ratios were four to one or six to one, depending on the shift and availability of staff. We insisted that one of us stay in the room with Scott. We were not looking for special treatment. All we wanted was to be allowed to sleep in the chair in the corner of his room. It was not an easy argument to win, but we did. Mike stayed that first night. On arriving early the next morning after getting everyone off to school, I met a friend, the superintendent of the high school my children attended, waiting in the hallway. He looked uncomfortable, even more than I expected. Dick had been in to visit us before and was well aware of Scott's condition, the look on his face told me something else was wrong. Without speaking to him, I ran down the hall to find Mike, who was busy trying to expedite a transfer for Scott back to an intensive care unit; this time, it would be pulmonary intensive care. He had developed a blood clot overnight and pneumonia as well. In less than two weeks, we had become very astute at reading the monitors, checking for signs of distress, and anything else that was out of the ordinary.

UMass Medical saved Scott's life more than once. The hospital was superb. The expertise and the compassion were excellent, but when someone is unable to speak or to articulate pain in any way, they need to have someone to advocate for them. My son would not be here today if Mike had not spent the night.

The transfer occurred. Scott's new home was now the seventh floor pulmonary intensive care unit. The pneumonia caused an extremely high temperature. Scott was spiking at 105 degrees. We were told that he needed cooling blankets, but that none were available for this seventh floor unit. We pushed for someone to get blankets from another unit, we had noticed some on the fourth floor from earlier in the week. The thought that these blankets could not be lent out to neighboring units was unthinkable, especially since my son's life was on the line. The matter was resolved within a few minutes, but not without much ado.

The impression we got from much of the staff those first few days in our new intensive care was that the battle was over and we had lost. He was not going to make it or at least not with any quality of life. We actually had one young intern tell us just that. He was not giving us odds, he was downright telling us that Scott would never have any quality of life again. I remember thinking to myself, "You're not much older than Scott, how much can you really know?"

What bothered us more was that he just made these off-handed remarks in front of Scott. If there was ever a chance that coma patients can hear and understand what is going on, this cocky intern just handed him a death sentence.

We needed to make the doctors and nurses on this floor understand that this young man was going to live. They needed to feel it as we did. They needed to know that he would be strong, intelligent, and living a life again one day. Then and only then would they give it their all. His life was worth saving.

It's funny even today all these years later, certain behavior will bring back the memories of this ordeal. Today, life is good, back to normal, and yet certain simple actions bring me back to this nightmare. While mindlessly strolling through the grocery store the other night, my husband pushing the cart, I walked aimlessly, not interested in making any purchases (never grocery shop on a full stomach). I found myself deliberately walking on the center of every other linoleum tile on the floor, carefully making sure not to touch the cracks of any of the tiles. I did this for no reason, other than sheer boredom. Last time I walked this way, it was so deliberate. The hospital corridor, outside the ICU, and scared to death. The procedure was placement of an IVC filter; this would hopefully prevent future blood clots from hitting Scott's lungs. Comparatively speaking, this was a simple procedure, but not for me, not in my mind. I kept thinking he made it through so much, and now this is going to kill him. For over an hour, I paced the floor, making sure to avoid the cracks. I couldn't stop. I remember thinking I had to keep moving, reasoning it out wasn't an option.

About twenty-three days were spent in pulmonary ICU. The first two weeks were grim. Scott's condition went from bad to worse. He survived the fall, barely, but now, there were so many more problems, new problems. While still in a coma, he developed MRSA (methicillin-resistant staphylococcus aureus), pneumonia, Rigors (severe chills and trembling caused by extremely high temperature), and had fevers spiking at 105 degrees. His lungs were filled with fluids, he was continually being suctioned, and fighting against blood clots on a daily basis.

Our days were filled and exhausting. I recall exercising Scott's arms and legs through repetitive movement. We were told that this would help in preventing more blood clots. Our instructions were that twenty leg lifts at a time would be appropriate, so we did one hundred, stopping only to suction his tracheal tube, wipe his eyes, or pray. Mike and I, my son Michael, and Scott's girlfriend Jill became all too comfortable with suctioning and cleaning his trach.

Jill had been dating Scott for a little more than a year when this tragedy struck. She was strong and beautiful, a Sandra Bullock lookalike. Growing up with five brothers, she was quite comfortable in our family. But it wasn't until this tragedy struck that we knew the depth of her strength.

WAKE ME UP WHEN SEPTEMBER ENDS

Scott

My next memory was of my brother, Michael pinching me so incredibly hard. From all medical reports, I was still in a coma, but the memory is vivid. Picture this, two hundred pounds of muscle putting all his energy into pinching your chest with a massive amount of adrenaline working for him at the same time. I was trying to stop him, trying desperately to get my arms and legs to move, but it was like a communication breakdown. "Stop, Michael! Stop, Michael!" kept repeating through my head but I couldn't move or say a thing. I kept screaming, but in reality, I was silent as a mute. I had no idea where I was or why I was here or what was going on. It was as if I was getting a "No Service" signal, like the kind you get on a cell phone.

Months later, I learned that my mother and Michael, would routinely pinch my arm and chest in an effort to wake me up, a trick they learned from one of the physicians. That never became the practice with the rest of the family. Not sure if that makes them more or less compassionate!

YOU RAISE ME UP

Linda

Through all of this, on October 10, Scott finally emerged. I was down the hall in the waiting room talking with Bob and Sean Conley and Bob's wife Phyllis. These people were business associates that became close friends. I have always been one who seems to blur the lines between personal and business, but that was just fine with me.

Mike was in the room with Scott. As Scott opened his eyes, however slightly, he could tell our Scott was there. He told Scott he loved him and he had to get Mom. He started calling me from the other end of the hall. I could hear his voice echoing such a rush of emotion, this had to mean good news. As I turned and rushed down the hall from the Conleys, I remember feeling as though my legs were not going to hold me up. I couldn't get to him fast enough.

I saw him. His body fragile. He had been lying motionless for twenty-three days, but for that short time for those few minutes, all I could see was my Scott. I could look into his eyes and I knew he was in there, *we knew*. This was the beginning, this was the answer to my prayers. This moment has been emblazoned in my soul forever.

One never knows how they will react when emotions take over. You react because of instinct, compassion, or so many other emotions we are not even able to articulate.

My reaction was one for the books. I hugged and I kissed him and told him how much I loved him, how much he needed to be strong, we needed to be strong and we would all be okay. Then I put him to work. He had rested for twenty-three days. Time to work. He was unable to speak, unable to move his arms, legs, or neck, but he could move his fingers on his left hand, very slightly. That was enough.

We started quizzing him. I told Scott I would put my hand in his left hand and I wanted him to move his fingers, squeeze my hand as best he could when the correct answer was given to each question. It was my way of staying the course. Through all of this ordeal, I took a very narrow view of things. Scott was going to recover, fully, he was going to be all right. I could not cope with thinking outside of this realm. It was my survival. So it was then, we began. What college do you attend? After naming fifteen or so Massachusetts colleges, I named Becker, Scott squeezed. I was ecstatic, we continued. I held up a pizza box, left over from someone's lunch, and quickly demanded. What am I holding; McDonald's, Burger King, Arby's, or Papa Gino's? The squeeze came at the right time and so did my tears.

We did this for what seemed like an hour, but in reality, it was only minutes. Scott fell back into a state of semi-coma, but we knew now, what I had always known, he was healing, truly healing. His awakening was a benefit in another sense as well. As he was still in ICU, the staff witnessed his brief state of consciousness. They saw, as we did, that there was real hope that this young man would live again, not just exist.

From that day on, there was something very different about Scott's treatment on the seventh floor. It is human nature to be more committed when there is hope. We were no longer alone.

Scott

The "squeezing the hand conversations" went on for days, but a particular conversation that I will always remember went something like this. Michael and I were alone in the room. I could tell this by the silence and opening my eyes for just a few seconds at the beginning of his stay. I remember him speaking with what sounded like tears in his eyes. He told me that I absolutely had to survive because he would never be complete without all five Maloneys. He needed me to be the brother that always pulled Jen's pony-tail, wrestled with Jason, and teased our youngest brother Kyle. He wouldn't be content until I stood there at the altar as Best Man at his wedding.

Linda

Hours turned to days, and the days to weeks. Scott's emersion from his comatose state was amazing, but watching him lying there so still, often times in a semi-coma type of condition was an emotional roller coaster for all of us. I would sit next to Scott and tell him everything, everything I was thinking. In the back of my mind, my thought was that even when Scott was at his weakest, he would keep on fighting. If not for himself, then for us. I knew he loved us that much! It was while speaking to him one afternoon, while he seemed alert enough to understand my words, I prompted him to respond. After my earlier tests with him regarding the questions of what college he was attending, which fast food chain makes which food, I had to know one more thing. We had been told by so many professionals that an injury such as Scott's can often times change the core of the person, their personality. He could awaken, fully awaken to be totally different, someone we know longer knew. I was so scared. I had to know if this limp lifeless body lying there was still Scott. I asked him just that, thinking back I was probably putting enormous pressure on him, but oh well, hindsight is always twenty-twenty. So I insisted, "Scott, give me a sign to show me you are you, something you and I will know and understand."

Since Scott had been able to squeeze his left hand, our conversations continued with 1 squeeze for A, 2 for B, 3 for C and so on. Scott would pause in between words. He began with "LUV" finishing with "EM" This was it! No more testing, I was good. This was a great day! Scott always used the term "luvem" rather than love you. All through high school and college, didn't matter his mood. As a teenager, he might be leaving the house, upset about something or someone, didn't matter, we always heard the "luvem" as he was leaving. It was my way of knowing everything's right with Son #2.

THE BOYS OF FALL

Linda

The fall of 2004 was a time of change for many. The Patriots were lining up for Super Bowl stardom, the Red Sox won the World Series, and on the same day that Scott emerged from a coma, October 10, 2004 Christopher Reeves (Superman), after an excruciating battle of his own, died. Billboards sprang up all over the area. Underneath his name were the words: *Strength, pass it on.* I remember the irony I felt at that time.

My daughter Jen, only eighteen, had, just a few months before this nightmare occurred, applied to Assumption College for admission, part of the process is to give the college a writing sample. This was her essay relating to an earlier, difficult time in Scott's life. Scott had no knowledge of this essay until it was read to him months later at UMass Medical.

College Essay

I have met Superman. The cultural icon that has captured audiences of all ages for many years is not so out of reach. The Man of Steel—the incredible being that never ceases to have courage in the face of the worst opposition—grew up in the small, quiet town of Plainville, Massachusetts.

The teenage years are the ones where friendships begin and trust bonds are formed. To miss out on such years could easily break any human spirit. As human beings, we crave social contact and depend on friendship. With the previous validated by one and all, I can say that one cannot imagine, without much difficulty, a worse situation than having been stripped of their early developmental years. Such was the case for my second oldest brother Scott. Struck down in his twelfth year by an unknown genetic disease that tends to run in my mother's family, Scott transformed in a mere month from being an avid athlete to having his only means of transportation being carried or by wheelchair. His condition was so bizarre that some of the very best doctors in Boston thought he was just "faking it." His spirit could have, and probably should have been broken in the two years, he had no choice but to hope that normalcy would return just as quickly as it left. But his spirit never did. My brother is the most resilient and rather simply amazing soul I have encountered. My brother is my Superman.

For years while growing up, Scott and I fought constantly. Now I feel nothing but awe and inspiration for him. His debilitating sickness taught me to never give up. Without speaking a word, my

Superman showed me that you needn't be able to leap buildings in a single bound to be revered, for he did no such thing and yet he is still revered and respected by me and all others.

My Superman taught me just how truly amazing the human spirit is. When some of the most intellectual minds in the world of medicine told him there was no hope, Scott defeated these "Villains" and won his battle. As the true identity of Superman lay undiscovered, so too did the incredible courage my brother had every day. Through his courage, I learned what it meant to be humble, through his two-year ordeal, I learned patience and through his greatness in recovery I learned what life is all about. My Superman gave me the greatest gift of all. He instilled in me the appreciation for everything that is taken for granted.

Jen Maloney

During those days on the seventh floor, every hour seemed like a new battle for Scott. MRSA was one of his biggest obstacles. It is a bacterial infection that is immune to most antibiotics. It is a real danger for patients with long-term hospital stays whose resistance is already down due to illness or injury. MRSA slowly attacks your immune system and can be fatal. The drug used to fight this infection (vancomyacin) is almost as dangerous as the infection itself.

We made friends during our stay. Mercy, the woman who prayed for him the night he was injured, shadowed us throughout his hospital stay. She would come by to check on Scott and his family. Those acts of kindness are never forgotten. I still save the letter she wrote to me in the corner of my wallet, all these years later.

10/08/04 — 0530am

Hello Linda,

How are you today? I came by to see Scott but didn't want to wake you up.

I am still believing and praying for "God's grace and mercy" I hope your family is okay otherwise. May God continue to be your strength in this trying time. God bless you and yours in Jesus's Name.

Mercy Essien

ONE DAY AT A TIME

Linda

When tragedy hits, coping is key, tunnel vision was my only way of coping. We were told so many times of the pitfalls...I knew them. We educated ourselves, we had to, but sometimes, the big picture was just too damn big. We had to win one battle at a time.

DON'T STOP BELIEVIN'

Linda

On October 20, Scott was discharged from UMass Medical Center and taken by ambulance to a local rehabilitation hospital, a mid-size rehabilitation center on the outskirts of Boston. There were other rehabs with bigger names and stronger reputations, but after interviewing with staff and touring the facility, we felt our choice was a better fit. The idea of choosing rehabs out of state was not an option for us. We had to be near Scott, all of us. Each of us felt, whether right or wrong, that our love, our help, and our constant focus on his recovery was as much a part of what was essential for him as the rehab itself.

This rehab seemed to broadcast that very thought. Their staff spoke about family involvement. I remember seeing posters on the walls in the corridors stating that the "TEAM" approach is our methodology; patient, family, and staff together can make a difference.

The morning we were to leave Mercy came by again. This time it was to say good-bye. She told me that our son would be okay and that he would walk again. She would continue her prayers. I thanked her repeatedly and so wanted to hug her, but something held me back, I felt that I had to stay strong. If I hugged and let my guard down, I would melt, collapse into something that we had no time for now.

The first few days in our new surroundings were positive. I remember the first time I saw the aides lift Scott in what is known as a Hoyle lift up onto a gurney in order to bathe him down the hall. It was the saddest sight and yet I felt elated. This was another baby step, but it was a step. Every day if we just take one step forward, we could bring him back. This is what we told ourselves. Some days it was easier to believe than others, but it was the only way I could make it through each day. I couldn't go outside the tunnel, if I allowed myself to think anyway other than full recovery, I wouldn't be strong enough for Scott, for me, or for my family.

The night after the accident when Scott held on to life by a thread, Mike and I found a quiet place in an empty hallway away from everyone. We sat on the floor, held each other, and cried. I remember Mike pleading with God, probably the first time he had spoken to him in years, asking him to spare his son and take his life instead. Just let him live, we'll sell the house, the practice, and anything else and take care of him forever.

God answered our prayers, he was going to survive, and I was already asking for more. Alive is not good enough, we need Scott back all the way.

That is how we dealt with each day. As the days and weeks passed, my friend Dick visited again. This time, it was at the rehabilitation center rather than the hospital. As a former school committee member, we had become friends and he was trying to console me. I told him to take a look at Scott. He was doing much better. He hugged me, patted me on the back, and without uttering a word, somehow got his message across. I knew what he was intimating. He was sure I was setting myself up for a fall. That in not facing reality, I would later be crushed. No words were spoken, but I knew. I hugged him, stared back, and assured him, "Scott is getting better."

During this nightmare, Scott had the constant support of his family and friends. He also had the love and undying devotion of his girlfriend Jill. She was young, only twenty, but had the wisdom and compassion of someone three times her age. She was one of six children and the only girl. I assume that this was why she had a toughness and strength that was unmatched. Aside from her beauty, we quickly realized what Scott found so amazing in her.

Christmas Eve 2003, long before any visions of this ordeal, Jill was at our house. Mike and I watched her react to our oldest son, Michael and knew then that she was something special. We had this short-lived tradition of playing musical chairs on Christmas Eve. It was originally planned for the little guys left in the family and a preempt to gift giving, but rapidly became a silly ritual for

the teens and young adults. Jill and Michael were compet-
ing for the win with a few others. They wound up vying for
the same chair and Michael, with his overzealous sense of
competition, pushed her ever so slightly in order to take the
chair. She pushed back, not so slightly, sat down, and with
a smirk, snickered, "I have five brothers, I don't think so."
We knew then that she was the right fit for this family. We
later came to find out that this silly game gave us a glimpse
of the real determination this young woman had.

The hours were like days and the days like weeks. The
rehab seemed to be reneging on their commitment to
"teamwork." As time passed and Scott's family persisted in
their round the clock care for Scott, we became more of an
annoyance than a part of the team to some of the hospital staff. Our daily overnighters with one family member
that were so welcome for the first few days were dissuaded
quickly. The extra bed in his room was removed by the staff.

An evaluation was scheduled for Scott. It was standard procedure that roughly two weeks after admittance to
the rehab, the lead physiatrist would sit with the patient,
go over medical records, and speak with the family to give
a long-term prognosis. We were told repeatedly that the
doctor on this case was one of the best in his field. Mike
and I waited for this day, as a young child would count
the days preceding Christmas. With all the talk we had
heard at the hospital, I had imagined this man to be our
savior. This was totally against character for both of us, we

question everything and put our faith in those only once we felt they have earned it. As it turned out, we should have stayed the course. Evaluation day arrived. The doctor was several hours late and met with Scott for less than five minutes. When he finally sat down with us to discuss our son's future, it took us just a short time to make our own diagnosis. He was discussing the wrong patient. When I disagreed with him about a symptom that he mentioned, that you need not have a medical degree to understand and told him that he was mistaken as to Scott, he glimpsed at the file on his lap and asserted that yes, he was talking about the wrong patient. He had the wrong file, then began a dissertation on quite a few generalities about patients with TBI. I was stunned, heartbroken, and furious all at the same time. We had awaited this precious visit, and it meant nothing to him.

Later that evening, I tried replaying the afternoon's ordeal, trying to rationalize and reason out why this would happen. After all, I was a professional, and yet on occasion, I have gone into a meeting unprepared and tried to bluff my way through it. But this was different, this was our son and our world. This was very different.

Scott

Not being able to communicate your basic human emotions is very trying. There are no words to explain the helplessness that I felt. When one feels sudden intense pain, human instinct tells us to immediately squeeze the region (just ask anyone who has missed the nail and hammered their own thumb), or when you don't understand a concept, you (a) ask a question to clarify or (b) the confused expression on your face can ask the question without using the actual words. I could do neither. I was emerging, waking up slowly, and trying to let others know. On more than one occasion, I tried so hard to convey a question or get across a statement that took what seemed like hours to interpret. When you take into consideration the lack of patience I have (as well as my family), the phrase "extremely frustrating" would be a major understatement. A prime example of needing patience is the following chronicle:

As previously mentioned, Michael had traveled much of the world and had backpacked many continents, making friends in hostels, airports, and bus stations. I would later find out that on one adventure (in Japan), he found himself needing a clean shirt, purchasing a blue polo with the word "Nippon" written in small letters on the top of it. He happened to wear this old blue shirt to the rehab. I spent what seemed to be an eternity spelling out the words, "What's Nippon?" No one knew what I was talking about and didn't seem to notice Michael's shirt. At that time, I was unable to even point at the shirt to explain my thinking. That question was not put to rest until a nurse walked in, heard my family, pointed to the shirt, and said it means Japan. I later came to find out that my folks were not only as frustrated as I was with trying to communicate, but they were also worried that I was unable to understand or make sense of things (since Nippon meant nothing to them). So the nurse's remark was a win on two levels.

VOICES THAT CARE

(October 2004)

Scott

Around this time, I began hearing something on the television. I remember the voices of the late-night trio. I never decided which one of the big two, Leno or Letterman, I liked better and my family knew this, which made them flip from channel to channel for me. What was good was the fact that there was no competition for the slot after Leno, which belonged to Conan O'Brien. I could recognize Conan, Jay, and Dave's voice because I often fell asleep in my dorm room to their shows as most college kids did. Hearing those three voices was not out of the ordinary. What was out of the ordinary was to hear the voice that I recognized as soon as I heard the first note. None other than Steven Tyler of Aerosmith singing the National Anthem acapella, just him, a harmonica and those unforgettable vocal chords (can ya tell I'm a big fan?). Just then I realized what was happening in Boston, specifically Fenway Park, the World Series.

Friends and family were telling me that I would be home before I knew it, well now I was starting to know it, and still, I wasn't going home anytime soon.

The Red Sox and the Patriots were constantly in the background but the 2004 Presidential election took control of the airwaves also. I prided myself on voting the person, not the party, but my Republican conservatism, was often overshadowed around the dinner table. With the exception of my dad, I came from a fairly liberal family. I recall my grandmother getting an absentee ballot for me. This was to be my first time voting in a presidential election and it mattered. She knew it. She held my hand as I squeezed out the name B-U-S-H. I later learned that the four registered Democrats in the house were unable to vote since they spent the entire day at my bedside. So in a way, I voted five times for Bush, you're welcome W!

My days and nights at the rehab, those that I can remember, were a roller coaster of emotions. Hope and despair would encompass me within minutes of each other. Here I was, a twenty-one-year-old in the prime of my life, someone who was voted MVP of my college cross-country team, someone who could bench press two hundred thirty-five pounds a few months ago, and someone who had run the Boston Marathon three years in a row. Now my greatest achievement, was being able to squeeze the fingers of my left hand.

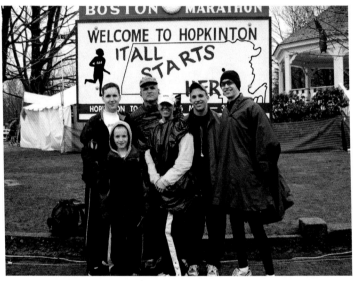

Boston Marathon
2007

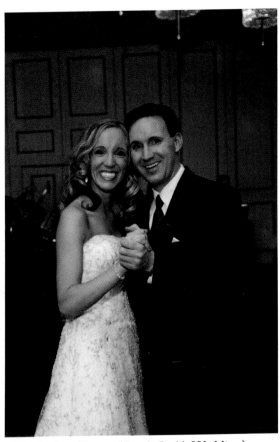

Sibling Dance (Jen & Josh's Wedding)
January 2011

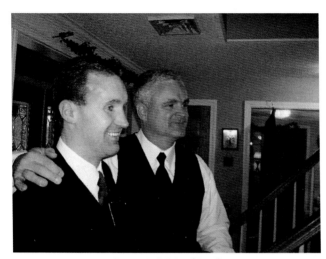

Scott & Mike (Dad)

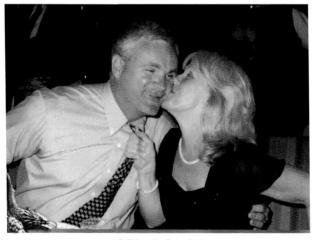

Mike & Linda

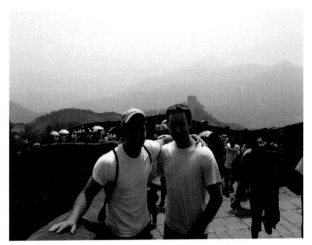

Scott & Jason - Great Wall of China
Summer 2011

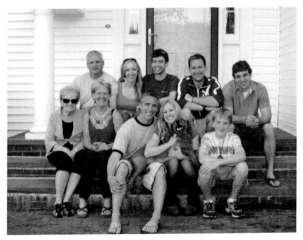

Family Picture

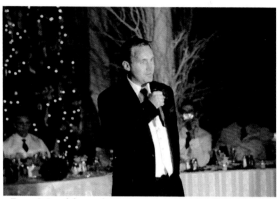

Best Man Toast (Michael & Johnna's Wedding)
December 2011

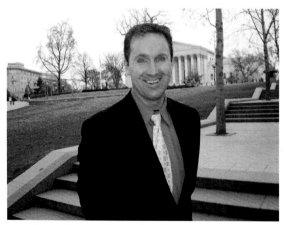

Brain Injury Awareness Day on the Hill
Washington DC
Spring 2012

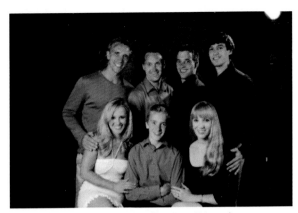

Family Cruise (Sibling Photo)
Summer 2012

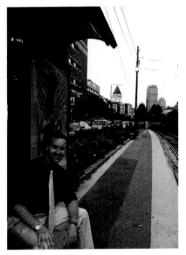

Riding the Green Line (Boston)
Summer 2013

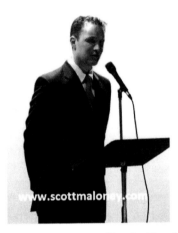

On the Road / Speaking

THE LONG AND WINDING ROAD

Linda

The days and nights became one long uninterrupted stay. The changes were marked only by the change in the nursing care and the noticeable change on weekends when physical and occupational therapy were discontinued. This allowed patients to spend more time with their families. We did not need nor desire the quiet time. We needed to push and keep on pushing. On warmer days, we would take Scott outside in the garden, anything for a change of scenery. He needed to wear a helmet at all times when not in bed, for he was still awaiting surgery to replace his skull. This could not be done until the swelling in his brain had stopped.

During this time, Scott had a trach and a feeding tube, was strapped into the wheelchair, wore a helmet, and was attached to monitors to keep track of his oxygen levels, so taking him outside in a wheelchair was no easy task. He was unable to speak, and since for most of his stay there, he was in a semi-coma type of state, unable to communicate in any way. But it seemed that just when we hit bottom, when we were at our most vulnerable, Scott would give us a sign. Anything small, we would take it. During his semi-lucid hours, we would rejoice and work that poor young man to death. Showing pictures, listening to music (Aerosmith being his favorite), writing on a white board, and getting a yes or no response. Our favorite way, our only way, of communicating was by holding Scott's hand and having him squeeze when we got to the letter that spelled the word to the question he was asking. It was fine for a question or two. But just like the physical therapy, the Maloneys pushed. One or two questions wasn't enough, all of us would keep talking, wanting Scott to be a part of the conversation. One time, he squeezed out the words: "Stop please." This would make our day worthwhile. This was all any of us needed for today, but tomorrow or the next time Scott was awake and aware, we needed a little more. This was the way we rationalized.

In cases of traumatic brain injury, all areas of the body can be affected. Except for his TBI, Scott had only minor injuries and yet was left unable to move. His right side was hit the hardest. He was burdened with something referred to as tone or "spasticity." The neurons in the brain misfire, causing the muscles to react too intensely at times caus-ing whatever extremity is affected to become stiffened and stone like. In those early days, the tone was extremely intense and affected both legs and his right arm.

Monday morning came and with that some good news, the swelling in his brain had decreased enough and Scott was scheduled for surgery to replace his skull. The whole family was elated. This would be a milestone in his recovery. Two weeks more, we couldn't wait! The surgery was scheduled, or was it? It turned out the rehab was not the only entity to cause us grief. The insurance company did their part as well. There was a glitch in this otherwise excellent coverage. Since Scott was still a full-time student in college when the accident occurred, he was covered under Mike's medical plan, but here's the glitch. About a week before the surgery was to occur (surgery to replace his skull), we got a call from our insurance company. It seemed they couldn't cover this procedure. It was another surgery and Scott was no longer a full-time student or a student at all, so no surgery. A kind of catch-22. People shouldn't have to deal with this type of craziness during good times, never mind during a crisis. After the first conversation with an insurance rep, we were told it was just an administrative matter, not to worry. It was merely a case of reclassifying Scott from a dependent student to a disabled dependent for insurance purposes. We were assured it would be taken care of within four to six weeks! *Postpone* the surgery until then! This didn't go over well. Such nonsense. "I can't do this anymore." I handed the phone to Mike, no, really, I threw it. After several lengthy conversations with the insurance rep and her boss and threatening to take our concerns to the press, the issue was resolved within twenty-four hours.

As Scott emerged further into our world, we had other issues to deal with. He became agitated at times; the swelling in his brain was going away, what a great thing, but as it did, what was so devastating was the shape of his head. It was enormously sunken and frightening to see. As this healing was taking place, so was Scott's ability to move his left side. He could now move his arm up to touch his face. This was great progress until one morning, he touched his head and the look on his face was that of pure fright. I grabbed his hand and told him that this was only temporary that the surgery was scheduled shortly. This calmed him somewhat.

Two weeks had almost passed. Surgery was to be tomorrow morning. All medications had been stopped in preparation for the surgery. The heparin drip discontinued. Surgery was to be at UMass Memorial in Worcester. The phone call came in. Surgery was postponed. About eight hours before what was to be our turning point, the operation was canceled. The surgeons were needed for an emergency that had just arrived. My intellect told me to understand that these things happen. After all, not all that long ago, Scott had been that emergency, but inside, I wanted to cry. We had to wait another two weeks.

Meanwhile at the rehab, we were not making any lasting friendships. Scott, still not himself, had tried on occasion to pull his tracheal tube out. Although we were there constantly, we asked that Scott be given a mitt for his left hand;

in case we fell asleep, we didn't want anything to happen. Reacting was not enough. This was not an easy task. We were told that legal issues prevented the staff from restraining Scott. All we wanted was a mitt on his left hand, so he would not pull out the tube that was keeping him alive. He could not yet move his right side, so that was not a worry. The lawyer in all of us convinced them that for legal reasons this was an option.

It was a Saturday morning; no physical therapy or occupational therapy today. We went for a walk pushing Scott in his wheelchair through the rehab and down to the garden. Scott was doing even better. Somewhat alert and communicating with us through our usual methods. Talk was about the Red Sox and the World Series they were winning. We were planning the next surgery and talking of better times after that. After the garden, we went back to the room.

As we got Scott back into his bed, he seemed to be going downhill. He was grimacing in pain. His temp on the rise and his blood pressure going up. All signs pointed to something being wrong, more wrong than what had become the norm. We waited for the doctors to evaluate. Walter Laskey waited with us. Walter was one of those people who for whatever reason became a big part of our daily routine. He was our high school's wrestling coach. Michael and Scott had both wrestled through school and Jay was now a captain on the team. Walter often told us when our older guys were in school that if Michael had Scott's natural agility and Scott had Michael's determination, they would have been unstoppable. I remember praying that Michael could somehow transfer his determination to Scott because right now, he needed both.

Over the days, weeks, months, and even years of this ordeal, Walter became so much more than a great coach. He became a source of strength, a sounding board, and a true friend in every sense of the word. A fifty-year-old ponytailed, ball-cap wearing wrestling coach. Angels come in all sizes and shapes. He didn't need to stop his life for us, but he did. I was told that one of the other wrestling parents asked why he spent so much time with all of us. His response simply, "How could I not, they're in pain."

After waiting for what seemed like forever, we were told that Scott was fine. They seemed to take the spike in blood pressure as just another setback, the grimacing pain, more meds needed, and the fact that his right leg was swelling to twice its size as a small setback.

Although unable to speak, the pain on Scott's face was evident and his vital signs were out of control. We pleaded for a second opinion since the doctor evaluating was merely an on-call doctor because it was a Saturday, and she was totally unfamiliar with his case. We were not. We knew something had to be done. Eventually, we did get another opinion. This doctor insisted that Scott be rushed to an outside hospital for an emergency fasciotomy, a limb-saving procedure used to treat acute compartment syndrome. We were told later that it was an unfortunate risk from the procedure that was performed to relieve the tone (spasticity) in Scott's right leg.

More than eight hours after our initial observation and informing the staff of these changes in his condition, he was finally transferred by ambulance to Beth Israel Hospital. I left the rehab and boarded the ambulance with Scott. Mike was already on his way to get the car to follow. I turned to my mother who was waiting by the entrance to be picked up. It was dark after 8:00 p.m., and yet through the lights from the ambulance, I could see the fear in her eyes. After all this, would he make it? Mike and the kids were so exhausted and overcome with grief, would they even make it to the next hospital? That night, my world was crashing in again.

An orthopedic surgeon was called immediately. The fasciotomy was needed to remove the blood that had emptied in and around the muscles in his calve. We were told before going in to surgery that amputation might be necessary in order to save his life. They wouldn't know until they got inside.

The surgery was successful. Once again, he incredibly beat the odds. Our new home, at least for a short time, was Beth Israel.

I couldn't help but feel so betrayed by this rehab. I wasn't upset about the bleeding; that was a risk we took when we consented to the procedure. What so bothered me, what still bothers us, is the fact that we were ignored for hours. Minutes were crucial, and yet, we were ignored for hours. That afternoon, we were told to go home by hospital staff, that our family's presence was a hindrance to Scott's healing rather than a help. One staff member had the audacity to tell me that Scott had told him that he wanted us to leave. Scott, at the time, had no voice and didn't regain use of his vocal chords until months later.

Our time at Beth Israel was only a blip on the radar, but once again, medical professionals saved our son. The surgery on his leg was successful. Part of the procedure in the fasciotomy was to leave the leg open. The leg was sliced more like filleted, and left open for several days. This allowed all the blood to drain to prevent further complications. Loss of so much blood meant that Scott had to undergo several blood transfusions. Within one week's time, we were ready for the next round of surgery. Time to return to Worcester, only this time it was UMass Memorial, a hospital closely affiliated with UMass Medical. Scott was scheduled once again to have his skull replaced. He was brought by ambulance to the surgical intensive care unit, given a bed, and prepped for surgery the following morning. This was the third ambulance trip I would take with Scott. This time, his life wasn't on the line, so they allowed me to ride in back with him. Mike and the kids all followed behind us.

Things were on track, we knew it would not be postponed this time. We were right. The surgery went smoothly, no complications. It was three days before Thanksgiving and we were thankful. Scott still had a long way to go, but we felt as though he was emerging; however slowly, he was still emerging from this dark hole. His ability to breathe on his own was improving daily. The day after Thanksgiving, doctors removed the trach. Although still unable to speak, Scott's eyes said it all. He knew what was going on when they pulled the tracheal tube out. Not at all what I had expected, a doctor merely pulled it out while Scott was lying in his hospital bed, but he need not be able to speak to communicate his fear. He knew that the trach was his lifeline for months, and now, it was gone without much ado. His eyes said it all, and with his left arm (he still had no mobility on his right side), he grabbed my hand and squeezed as if to say help me. After a short time, Scott realized that he was able to breathe on his own and the look of panic on his face subsided.

We were told that he would be leaving the intensive care unit within a day or so and onto a regular floor. But this time we didn't fight it. We felt he was ready.

Saturday morning came and Scott was moved. Things were going well, so many people were in this Saturday. We all knew he would be coming home soon. We were not going back to that rehab. We couldn't do that, we almost lost him there. We would handle rehab at home and as soon as possible make a daily routine of outpatient rehab at Spaulding Rehabilitation Hospital in Boston. Mike and I decided that we would take advantage of every type of therapy possible, but when it was over, we would take Scott home every night.

That afternoon, there were a half dozen or so people in the room, it was a semi-private room, but no one was in the other bed, which allowed everyone to be more relaxed; while some visited in the room, others waited their turn in the waiting area. I recall that day so clearly. The whole family was there. Even though Scott couldn't speak, you could see his personality slowly emerging. The kids were all talking about TV shows they used to watch years ago, just being silly about nothing at all. They got the notion to get Scott's arm some exercise by playing basketball with the trash barrel in the room and some plastic cups they had been using. Each time he scored, they would move the trash barrel away by just a few inches. Our hope was growing. Monday, he would be coming home.

Afternoon turned into early evening, something was wrong. That personality that was emerging was no more. I saw it in his eyes. We all did; everyone that loved him could see that he was slipping away. It was and still is hard to describe, especially to those new nurses on this floor. They hadn't taken care of him before today and didn't know what to expect. Mike and I talked but only for seconds, something was very wrong and something needed to be done.

We talked to the charge nurse and told her what we knew to be true. She called the neurologist on duty (but the wait was too long for us). Desperate, I went downstairs to the ICU and the nurses that had taken such good care of Scott earlier in the week. I rang the buzzer on the locked door. One of the nurses, Pam Emmerling, approached me, coat in hand, and ready to leave for the night. I began to speak, explaining or perhaps rambling about the decline of Scott's mental status. She put her arm around me as we entered the elevator. I needed to let her know that I had not told anyone that I was going to the ICU for more help. I didn't know just how that might play out upstairs, stepping on toes and such. She grabbed my hand, looked at me, and said, "I just met you in the elevator and wanted to check on an old patient." She was so calm. When we got to the room, she saw as we did that things were not right, got a hold of the neurologist immediately, and with such ease and professionalism, convinced all that he needed an MRI immediately. The MRI indicated that Scott's brain was bleeding again, out of nowhere, all over again.

We would later learn that during the surgery when Scott's skull was replaced, it was evidently replaced so precisely that it caused pressure against his brain and caused the bleed to begin again. Pam waited with us during the MRI and continued to wait and push to hurry things up. But this time, Dr. McGillicuddy was not available. We were told the surgeon on call was incredible, and we had no choice, no time to waste. Within an hour, he was in surgery. Brain surgery again. Scott was strong, but I couldn't help but wonder just how much one body could take. We waited for hours, huddled again in a surgical waiting room, too scared to move, to talk, or even to think beyond the next few minutes. After what seemed like a lifetime, the doctor came in and told us Scott had made it through the surgery, he was alive. Seconds before, Jill had left the waiting room to walk the hallways. She couldn't sit any longer. Upon returning and hearing the news, as she stood speechless in the middle of the room, she collapsed, her legs bowed, and as she fell to the floor, she muttered, "Now I can rest." We would not know the outcome until Scott was alert enough to somehow communicate, but he was alive. Once more, we felt like we had just dodged a bullet. This couldn't keep up. Scott was not the only one running on empty. We all were. If not for Pam Emmerling, neither the MRI nor the surgery would have occurred so quickly. She saved his life.

YOU'VE MADE THIS A
CHRISTMAS TO REMEMBER

Linda

It was early December, signs of the holiday season were everywhere. But this year, our Christmas was going to be different. Our gift was that Scott was coming home. On the morning of the fifth, we packed up our belongings. Checking out and saying good-bye to those who saved my son's life was an emotional time. These nurses and doctors cared so much. We were given page after page of instructions on medications, procedures, and appointments.

The trip home was via ambulance. I was once again allowed to take the ride. Scott was still in such bad shape that Mike was uncomfortable driving him home. He was still unable to swallow, he received his nourishment through a G-tube, he was unable to speak, his vocal chords had been damaged, and it was anyone's guess if his voice would return. He was unable to move except for his left arm. He couldn't even roll over in bed, but he was breathing on his own, and each day, he was just slightly more alert than the day before, ever so slightly.

Watching Scott being wheeled into his own home in a gurney tugged and pulled at every emotion in me. He was where he belonged, he was home, and he was medically stable. This was a great victory. But as I watched the ambulance leave our driveway, I looked over at my family and knew that our fight was just beginning. We needed him whole again.

My brother-in-law Tom was a great help to us during Scott's transition to home life. Tom was the president of the local Lion's Club and as such able to provide us with so much of what we needed: hospital bed, commode, shower equipment just to name a few. This was just another example of what family really means. Tom told me he could get whatever we needed, for as long as we needed it, and he did. Months later, as Scott improved, when these items were not necessary household fixtures, I told Tom he could have his organization pick them up. I meant now, today. I needed them to vanish today. If we didn't need them, I didn't want them around. Again, my way of coping, I had to keep moving forward. He complied without a complaint. He reminds me of that once in a while, if I tell him he's being irrational about something silly. Our support system was incredible in all of this.

The first night at home was frightening. None of us got any sleep. We had moved Scott's bedroom down to the first floor. We knew we had to set up a system, but didn't know just how it would work. The first few weeks at home, we spent our nights on the floor of Scott's room, afraid that he would need us in the middle of the night and not be able to call for us. He had gone from a 190 pounds to 135, but it still took a lot to move him. He was almost like dead weight.

One of Scott's first trips after he came home was to his brother Jason's wrestling match at the high school. We brought him in a wheelchair; he was unable to hold his head up without help, his neck muscles had become so weakened, he couldn't speak, and he was able only to move his left hand, but he knew where he was and what was going on around him. I couldn't bear to see the pity in the eyes of so many, but we needed to keep his mind and body moving forward.

Jason's friends were there, their hearts broken as they greeted Scott. The last time they saw him, he would have wrestled them out on that mat and won. But it was clear every day to more and more people that he was returning. Dick Robbatt was there that night, and this time, he saw it. In the distance on the other side of the mat, I saw him. As he approached, he spoke to Scott, and as he raised his eyes to meet mine, he said you were right, I see it now.

It was at that moment I felt my heart swell, just like the Grinch in the Christmas cartoon. I really felt it. With that one statement I knew that others could see what I knew to be true, what I so needed to be true!

I'LL BE HOME FOR CHRISTMAS

Scott

I remember the day pretty well, December 5, 2004. Going against the advice of many, I was going home. My parents believed I would receive better care at home while going to a rehab daily as an outpatient. I was not afraid of dying anymore, but I was still scared. I felt like death was pursuing me (not only myself but others). I feared the death of a family member or close friend. I had been through so much, that I was afraid for those I loved. I had no idea of the emotional turmoil ahead of me.

Before my accident I weighed in at 190 pounds of muscle. Now I was down to 135 pounds of skin and bone. Jill joked that she would leave me if I got below 125 pounds (her weight). As I was wheeled out in the hospital bed, I remembered some advice I got years ago as a freshman in college on the soccer team. It was to give the international sign that you were going to be okay if you were ever injured on the field. Raising one hand in the air, giving the thumbs up, as they placed the stretcher in the ambulance. I made sure to give this signal, not only for those watching, but for myself as well.

The ride seemed long probably because I was awake and alert this time, connected only to a feeding tube. With an EMT driving and two paramedics in the backseat and my mother riding shotgun, I remember Kentucky Fried Chicken being talked about the whole trip home by one of the paramedics. This guy must have had some of the Colonel's blood in him because he kept bashing all of the other fast-food chains. Meanwhile, all I could think of was, I haven't had anything to eat in three months.

I'm home! I made it! I remember everything just as well as everyone else from this point on. I remember thinking that my parents might be questioning whether or not they should have brought me home so early after my injury. I wanted to let them know that things would get better. This was a good day. I, always the comedian, dragged my right foot in the wheelchair and headed for the refrigerator (still on a feeding tube). With the door open, I pointed at what I was looking for. I never liked cheese, but I always had fun with a trick I did with Sable, our five-year-old German Shepherd. Months before, what seemed like a lifetime ago, I would put a piece of cheese in my mouth and close my eyes. Sable would then leap up and grab the cheese from my mouth without touching me. So barely able to move my arm, I put the cheese in my mouth. Sable performed perfectly, while navigating around the feeding tube and the family members. I needed to make them laugh.

I fell asleep that afternoon as soon as my head hit the pillow. If nothing else was right, I was home and that was right. A sense of calm came over me.

I made it home to a hospital bed and a wheelchair. My parents slept on the floor in my room next to my bed, fearing they wouldn't know if I needed them in the middle of the night. I had to be carried in and out of the bathroom, unable to tend to my own needs. Modesty was not an option. As I recall, there were not too many options at all. I had to swallow my pride which is easier said than done. I had so much pride to swallow that I damn-near choked.

Christmas at the Maloney's was always a big event. Christmas Eve was always spent with my father's side of the family, Christmas morning with immediate family, and the afternoon with my mother's family. It was one continuous celebration filled with everything Christmas is about. This year was different, quiet, no visitors, except for Jill, no Christmas presents, and what I remember well was the fact that there was no Christmas music playing. It was kind of that bittersweet feeling you get when you just can't get ahold of which emotion you're feeling. But I was alive and home. That was my gift!

I'LL BE THERE

Linda

Scott was home now, facing new challenges for him and for his family. He would survive, but now, the struggles would be so different and a new one would unfold in front of us each and every day.

It was still early December. Scott had only been home a couple of days. My sister, Debbie, came by to see us, just as she had done so many times in the hospital and in the rehab. Debbie and I love each other so deeply and yet are polar opposites. We love each other, our children, and each other's children. Scott and my niece, Val, grew up more like twins than cousins, they were inseparable.

This particular day, except for Scott we were alone in the house, very unusual for that time. Scott had not tried to stand since his accident and I was anxious to get his life moving forward. I had what the physical therapists refer to as a gait belt. The hospital gave it to us when we left. The gait belt gets strapped around Scott and wrapped around those trying to support his weight. I wanted Debbie to help me lift Scott from his bed and walk down the hallway with him. She didn't want any part of it. She didn't want to be responsible if he got hurt. I still recall how vehemently she insisted that this was not a good idea. I begged her and told her that she had to help me, that we had to keep pushing him. Debbie is two years older than me, and with very different personalities, I was never able to talk her into too much. But that day was unlike so many others, she looked at me, I hadn't convinced her, hadn't talked her into anything, but she knew I needed this. What I remember most was the way she looked at me, in spite of her frustration, there was so much love and concern in her eyes. We stood up, Scott in the middle, as she mumbled, "If we drop him, I'll kill you!"

We live in a quiet neighborhood, in a small town between the outskirts of Boston and Providence. The house sits on a hill with a cobblestone type walkway leading from the driveway to the front door. There is a small stone wall at the foot of the walkway, and it wasn't until writing our story that I realized the significance of that wall and that walkway.

I used to go outside and sit on that wall and quietly pray to God to help us. Early in the morning or late at night, it didn't matter; when I felt at my weakest and most vulnerable, I would go outside at the foot of the walkway and pray.

In early December shortly after Scott came home, I recall running out for a quick errand. On the way back in the house, I dropped to my knees and prayed again for

God's help. I recall thinking was this really a prayer, because half of me felt that the only reason I wound up on my knees was because I felt to weak to walk anymore. This war was exhausting. Our front yard is thick with pine and oak trees, so I felt safe from the world; no one would see or hear me, for these few moments, while I desperately prayed for help.

As I mentioned, it wasn't until pulling this book together that I quite understood the significance of this spot. This later became the very spot where Scott first stepped from his wheelchair and later let go of his walker and took those first few steps alone.

Being on a hill, the walkway is on a slight incline, not the perfect place for one to try to resume standing or walking again, but it was our spot. As I pushed the wheelchair forward, I told Scott that I just wanted him to stand for a moment. He did, holding on nearly knocking the both of us down, but he did. Weeks later with the walker, I told him to try just one step without aid, and I would give it back to him after just one step. Scott had improved some at this point and was able to communicate without saying a word a resounding *NO!* After much ado, he took one step, then, another and another. The promise to give it back was not adhered to, but Scott knew me as well as I knew him and this came as no surprise. With these small steps came new possibilities. Tears swelled in our eyes that day, in the same place where I had fallen to my knees in prayer.

When tragedies such as Scott's strike, people are not prepared. Mike and I were no different. Through all of Scott's recovery, we made decisions, tried vehemently to sound self-assured, so as to give Scott all the reassurance that he needed. But every hour and every minute that went by, we were scared. We questioned every decision. Were we pushing too hard or not hard enough? We were told constantly by so many professionals that Scott only had so long to recover, and after that time, he would peak no more. A window of opportunity, some said six months, others a couple of years and still others (the minority) that declared there was no window that recovery was ongoing. In retrospect, we now know the latter was correct, what we believed all the time, but nonetheless, we had to push, what if we were wrong.

It was January and Mike still had not gone back to work. His head would not have been in it, and as a pilot, he needed to be focused at work. I worked for myself and had the luxury of having an office only a mile from home. The first day I went back to work for what was to be only a couple of hours. It turned out to be more like a few minutes. Mike called me on my cell. "Listen to this." Listen was the cry I heard. "Mom, Mom" in a raspy whisper was all I could hear, but I heard it. Mike heard it, and most importantly, Scott heard it. He was on his way. His voice was returning, still not ready to take the stage or wow his audience, that would come later. Baby steps.

Slowly, we tried to encourage our kids to return as much as they could to the routine that their lives once had. Before all this, Michael had been looking to buy a condo and move out on his own, so in January of 2005, he did just that. He found a place about ten miles away. The family loaded up the truck with furniture gathered as most young people do from relatives and friends who have too large a collection of their own. This was the way things were supposed to be. Our twenty-four-year-old son was moving out. But the everyday, relaxed feeling, disappeared abruptly as I watched Michael carry Scott up three flights of stairs to his condo. I needed to be strong, shrug off the depression that quickly consumed me and thank God he was alive. There's an old expression that goes something like this, "As much as things change, they always stay the same." Within weeks, Michael had moved back home and put his brand-new condo on the rental market. Michael's statement as he raced through the front door, "I need to be here, Scott needs me through his recovery."

It was also in early January when Scott began outpatient therapy at Spaulding. He went each day for physical, occupational, and speech therapy, three hours a day, five days a week. We were told that this would be the same schedule if he were enrolled in inpatient services, but after what we had been through at the other rehab, we were all more comfortable with returning home each evening. I'm not sure that there is any way that the professionals involved in these fields have any idea of the impact of their statements, the profound impact of a simple comment can be unforgettable. The first day we arrived for rehab, Scott was sitting in his wheelchair, looking helpless and beaten. The individual sitting behind the desk, routinely filling out forms and such, glanced up at the two of us and stated quietly, "It's only a mountain, only one mountain." He smiled and returned to his work, and yet almost ten years later, I still remember his face and his words. This man gave me such hope.

Within three weeks' time, Scott was on his way back to school, continuing the therapies, but on his way to his future.

STAND BY ME

Scott

It was January, or maybe February 2005, unable to walk, but my incredible, unflinching, stand-by-me brothers (I'm sure I wasn't so complimentary at the time) had me at the local YMCA. Still donning a feeding tube in the pool, I had to leave a T-shirt on in order to hide it. Michael and Jason probably, rightfully so, thought that the powers that be at the Y might not be happy with the idea of the feeding tube. Unable to speak, unable to swallow, I remember choking on the water. In retrospect, it was probably good for them that I couldn't speak at the time. If you guys are reading this now, thanks, I know I was not a cooperative participant.

BACK TO BECKER

Linda

Improvement continued, but sometimes so slowly that Mike and I would have to sit down, scrutinize events of the day or week to find the improvement. When you start all over again, it's a long road. It was about the third week of January, Scott and I were on our way home from therapy. Scott was speaking, only in whispers, but that was enough for then. As I merged onto the highway from the parking lot, Scott asked me to go in the opposite direction, toward Worcester. His voice was even softer than usual, kind of shaky as he mumbled the words, "I know it sounds crazy, everyone will think it is crazy, but I want to go back to school."

It was crazy! So what else do crazy people do? Crazy things! Calling Mike on the way to Becker was the first priority. Second semester classes were already underway, so Scott needed to convince the administration that he was able to take a class or two. A tough feat for Scott, since he was in a wheelchair, had minimal use of his arms, a voice barely audible, and a feeding tube (he was still unable to swallow). But he did it. Mentally Scott was back. His memory, quick wit, outgoing personality, and love of life, family, and friends...all still in tact. His eyes told the story and his smile denoted the thanks when they okayed him for classes. My thought was that the board allowed him back out of loyalty and compassion for an injured student, without the thought that he would ever graduate, but that didn't matter then. A win was a win!

Scott started back with two classes. After just a few weeks, he progressed from a wheelchair to walking or should I say hobbling into class. This was an uneasy feeling for Scott and my family, but the right thing to do and the right time to do it. The staff at Becker went above and beyond to make sure that Scott had everything he needed to start back to school. The faculty did so much, even though I'm sure some of them had their doubts as to what Scott or his parents were doing. His damaged vocal chords made it difficult for both staff and students to realize that it was his voice, not his comprehension, that was the problem. I would drive him back and forth, waiting in the lounge or in one of the professors' office who had befriended me while Scott was in class. I'll never forget Professor Dorsey. He was also an attorney, and Irish which he reminded me of all the time. Every morning I was there, he would tell a different freshmen student that it would earn them an A, if they could go get the two of us coffee and a muffin. He had a big family himself, knew my pain, and as such, had a corny joke to offer to brighten the mood. I looked forward to it. The cornier, the better.

Things were going well, Scott also enrolled in some online classes and, before we knew it, was back talking to the administration. Because Becker is a small school, and Scott was by no means a quiet guy, he was already well-known with these folks, long before the accident. This time he was convincing them that he needed to (walk) graduate with his class and finish the required credits over the summer. This was a harder argument to win, but the administration allowed him to walk across stage with the graduating class, under the stipulation that he would get his official college degree after successfully completing the summer courses.

Scott

It's funny how you remember the small details during big events. Class had already begun and I was the last one to enter (I used to like making an entrance). It was a small classroom with a dominantly male population as is customary in law-enforcement classes. As I was wheeled into my first class by another student, my thoughts ran rampant. Would they judge me for making such a stupid decision, pity me for who I am today, or both? Could I find the strength to put a smile on my face, as it took so much effort just to hold up my head? This was tough, tougher than I thought it would be. Then, as I poised myself for the stares and slowly arched my back, I heard it. "There he is!" followed by applause and sincere smiles. I vividly recall those first words. I recall the applause and the feeling of apprehension that, seconds before, was overwhelming me quickly diminished. The "forgotten semester" was no more. This was it. I was back, not what I expected for my last semester in college, but I'd take it.

GRADUATION DAY

Linda

Graduation day came, and what a day that was! Held at the DCU Center, the crowd was enormous. We were there so early that we were able to get seating in the second row. Between my family and Josh (Jen's boyfriend), Jill, Ben and my niece, Val, we nearly filled an entire row. We had one unexpected visitor attending the graduation. Her name was Pam Emmerling; she was one of the nurses who single-handedly saved Scott. Sometimes, actions truly speak louder than words. She had a husband and children of her own. She barely knew us and yet that Saturday in May she was there with us.

As they called the names of the graduates, my heart was racing. I was feeling every emotion imaginable, joy over this occasion, sadness for the year Scott had lost, and the struggles he had left to fight and scared that he was not stable and strong enough yet to walk across the stage without falling. Mike climbed the stairs on the other side of the stage to meet Scott. His embrace melted my heart. I truly have amazing children because they have an amazing father.

Scott

I remember the day I graduated from college, May 14, 2005, it was one of the happiest days of my life. Technically, I didn't officially graduate until the end of the summer to make up for the "forgotten semester," but I "walked" for my graduation, I took part in the ceremony. I still remember that day very well, everyone there supporting me. The Master of Ceremonies at every graduation always gives the same spiel, about how you should save your applause until the final name has been called ...yada yada yada...that rule is seldom if ever obeyed. Becker College is a small school and my graduating class was only a few hundred people. But despite Becker's size, my commencement was held at the DCU center, a large venue in downtown Worcester. I was already planning my walk across the stage. When my name was called, I did not want to limp, I did my best not to limp, but I'm sure trying to hide the limp made it even more noticeable. The man with the ominous voice started calling out the names, Shawn Lisee (loud applause), Matthew MacCormack (loud applause), then the voice paused for only a second and said, "Scott Edward Maloney," my memories are probably exaggerated a lot, but my recollection is that the eruption of applause was deafening. I'm pretty sure the uproar rivaled the same applause that was heard at Woodstock!

After the commencement, the Maloney entourage went out to lunch in Providence as all the Worcester area restaurants suitable for post-graduation lunches would most likely be overcrowded with so many Worcester area college graduations on the same day. We were at one of the many small Italian restaurants on Federal Hill when my brother Michael gave me an envelope, I opened it and inside I found a flight itinerary with a trip for two to Ireland. Michael and I were going to Ireland! I had completely forgotten that about a week before my accident we had planned a trip to Ireland. Obviously, that was forgotten by the both of us after the hell I put my family through...or so I thought. Michael remembered and gave me a printed itinerary for a flight from Boston to Dublin for early December 2005, giving me more time to recover.

JESUS TAKE THE WHEEL

Linda

Summer of 2005 brought more challenges. With every victory came a new challenge, one that you didn't even think of until the previous one was conquered. Mercy had warned me of this, the day we left the medical center. But that day I clearly remember thinking, that although I have placed this woman on a pedestal, and although I believe it was her faith in God and her prayers that were responsible for saving Scott's life, no matter how great she was, here she was wrong. "He will walk and talk again and every time you see him you will give glory to Jesus' name," then she took me aside and whispered, "But it will not happen as quickly as you think, it will TAKE TIME." You think I would have been ecstatic with a miracle, many miracles, but me being me, I needed to believe that it would be today. It turned out, she was right again.

Classes continued and I was still driving Scott back and forth to school. Everything was moving forward so quickly, much to the surprise of the rehab.

One day while driving home from classes, Scott asked me to pull over in the breakdown lane. I thought it was the typical guy reason to pull over in the breakdown lane and take a walk in the woods, but it wasn't. We were on the Mass Pike, a road very familiar to him. He asked me for the keys, *He wanted to drive the rest of the way home. I thought, he's ready, he can do this. God will take care, he wouldn't have brought us this far only to fail.*

As we began to pull out on the highway, I warned, "There's an eighteen-wheeler coming down the road, let him pass before you pull out." Scott's response without skipping a beat was "No way, I can make it." As he chuckled, but cautiously waited for the truck to pass, I felt a sense of calm come over me. This ridiculous comment made me relax, because this was my son...same as always.

Everyone everywhere that has grown up in a supportive family, traditional or otherwise, knows and understands how each member has their role within that family. Psychologists' research attribute birth order as being a primary factor to the character of an individual. I'm here to tell you that the mother's role is the toughest! She has to be strong, nurturing, and loving to her children, but when dealing with an adult who needs to get back not only physically but emotionally to where he was before, she needs to fight those very instincts, step back, and let him learn to fight again alone. It was a constant struggle within myself.

I still recall the first time Scott started driving on his own again. He went to pick up his brother at the train station about six miles away from home. He left the house, nervous but ready, much more ready than I was. I left about thirty seconds after him and walked, continually, incessantly, around the block, up and down the street, unable to stop, until I saw the car pull into the driveway.

THAT'S WHAT FRIENDS ARE FOR

Scott

Throughout my recovery, both in the hospital and at home my best friend, Ben came on weekly visits just to put a smile on my face, which is something he could do with ease. On one occasion, he went into my closet, picked up a baseball, and signed it "Barry Bonds" in front of me just to get me to smile, it worked. Throughout my ordeal, so many people played so many different roles. Ben's was to keep my spirits up the best he could and he did, at least for a while.

If you've made it this far into our story, you are certainly aware of my close network of faithful family and friends. A major paradigm of true friendship is the following story about Ben and his now-wife Judy. At the time of this tale, Judy was his girlfriend. About a year after my injury, I introduced Ben to an old friend of mine from high school, Judy. As a matter of fact, "Jude" and I went to our high school prom together. They started dating. While they were dating, Ben ran the Boston Marathon. Judy, Ben's mother, Terry, and I went to watch and cheer him on. At the time, my arm would lock up whenever exerting myself, even minimally, like a short walk. It's called spasticity. My arm locking up would cause immense throbbing pain, but what was worse was the distortion. It would tighten up so much it looked like I was carrying a rifle under my sleeve. I'm not sure which bothered me more, the pain or the embarrassment. We began to walk toward Cleveland Circle, a popular place to glimpse the marathoners as they began their last stretch of the race, hoping to see Ben. Like clockwork, my arm locked up. Judy noticed. As any great friend would do, she grabbed my arm and held my hand and made it appear as though we were a young couple walking arm-in-arm to watch the race. No one was the wiser, though it probably raised Terry's eyebrows a bit!

My friends come in all shapes and sizes. Walter Laskey is one of them. Small in stature, but a heart bigger than most and a grit that is unsurpassed. He was capable of "pushing your buttons" to get you motivated and did so. He was my high school wrestling coach, but much more than that. After my injury and initial rehab, he was there to push my buttons again. He spent the spring and summer of 2005 working with me, bringing me back. Walter could always tell when my head wasn't in the game and would let me know it in no uncertain terms. One hundred percent and no less was his attitude; emotionally, I was just not there, but he wouldn't give up.

One hot, humid August afternoon, Walter and I were going on a run. We met up at Foxboro Center and ran,

I use that term lightly, to an outlying farm just a couple of miles away. My vision was blurred by the droplets of sweat pouring down my face and the stench of my own perspiration was tough to take. But worse than all that was the knowledge that I did not run as I once did. My gait was shaky and awkward and my right arm tightened up (spasticity... again). As I made it toward the entrance to the farm down a long driveway, I knew I could finish and I knew why. Walter was one of those people that push you so hard. You would do whatever it was he wanted of you, not just to prove him wrong, but to shut him up. In my book, Herb Brooks, Bill Belichick, and Vince Lombardi take a backseat to Walter Laskey's coaching. He's a never give up kind of guy.

WHEN I WAS YOUR MAN

Scott

Jill was hands-down the best girlfriend a young man could ever ask for, especially considering the life circumstances I put her through, I went from being:

A man who never shed a tear ... To a crybaby.

Someone with all the confidence in the world ... To having no confidence.

Not relying on anyone ... To a Mama's boy.

Having a hard body ... To flabby and out-of-shape.

Someone who put his girlfriend at the center of his world ... To someone that gave her a supporting role.

Jill had transferred from Keene State College (Keene, New Hampshire) to Nichols College (Dudley, Massachusetts), which was just a few minutes from her home. She did this for only one reason, to be closer to me. It seemed that no matter how hard I pushed her away, she would pull me toward her. I cried like a baby, called her names, and acted like someone with the maturity level of a twelve-year-old. But she stayed by my side until I pushed one time too many.

Physically I was improving, but emotionally, I was plummeting. With healing came the knowledge and understanding of just how badly injured I was. With that also came the uncertainties and insecurity that I would ever become as Toby Keith would say, *"As Good as I Once Was."*

I tried as hard as I could to distance myself from everyone that ever meant anything to me. I didn't want their pity; I didn't want them to see my weakness. I was spiraling downward and continued to push people away. I even pushed away that beautiful young woman, the one who meant so much to me, the one who stood by my side. I couldn't help myself, but I did. I pushed so hard that...I lost her.

I pushed others as well, my family, my mother and father, and all of my siblings. As hard as I pushed them away, they all pushed back even harder. Thank goodness for my family, my stubborn family. If they had not been there to fight for me, I wouldn't be here today. They would not leave me behind.

CELEBRATE

Linda

September 18, 2005, marked the one-year anniversary. We all went out to dinner that night, kind of a bittersweet celebration, marking another milestone. Things were changing, normalizing.

Michael had moved to New York over the summer. He was working in marketing and finishing his third year of law school, commuting back to Boston a few nights a week for school. Jen, in her second year at Assumption, decided that she had no interest in living in the dorms and remained a commuter student throughout the remainder of her college years. Jason was now a senior in high school, looking forward to graduation and his college years ahead. Kyle was in third grade. This year had been a whirlwind for him, too, young to fully understand the tragedy that his family has endured, yet old enough to see their pain.

Mike and I were back to work. Since my office was so close to home, it was easy to come back and forth whenever needed. It was easier too, because throughout this ordeal I was fortunate to have a paralegal who had the professionalism and dedication to keep my office running when it was the last thing on my mind. Lori Seavey and I met about a year before Scott's accident and she quickly became a staple in the office. What I didn't know then was that as time passed she would become so much more than a valued coworker. She became a forever friend. She became family, in every sense of the word. Our paths were meant to cross.

Although physically Scott had improved so much, emotionally, he was a mess. Every day he seemed to get stronger, but mentally, he was spiraling downward. It seemed that he was becoming aware of just how close he had come to the brink of death, to the year he had lost, and the knowledge that in spite of the fact that he had come so far, he still had miles to go before he was where he needed to be, where he wanted to be, healed and whole again. His confidence had been shattered so deeply.

Before all this, Scott was a very confident young man, full of life. He wanted so to be that person again, now. Right now. He was tired of waiting. I understood. Patience did not come naturally for any of us. It was a virtue that we had to learn.

For a while after Scott started doing more, he worried more. He became nervous about driving, what if I get hurt again? He was not only fearful for himself, but for those he loved. He became fearful about everything. One day while taking groceries out of the backseat of the car, he tripped on something next to the car. In doing so, he hit the backseat with his shoulder and the side of his head. He panicked. Really panicked. "What if" was all he could get out. The "what ifs" were taking over his world. He started pushing everyone away his parents, his siblings, and his girlfriend. This was all so new to us, we didn't know how to respond.

Shortly after Scott had returned home from the hospital, Jill came by. She spent every extra moment with him. We let Jill borrow Mike's car temporarily as he was still not back to work and she needed something reliable for the hour and a half commute from her home. She had become a fixture in our home, and we welcomed that.

Early one night, it was still wintry outside, but we had burgers on the barbecue for dinner. While we were bringing food inside from the back porch, she stopped me, pulled me aside, and said, "I just need to know that Scott will be able to make me laugh again, everything else I can handle." All those months later when Scott pushed her away and she needed someone, I wasn't there for her. She deserved more than that; we had grown to love her and yet we let her disappear from our lives as though she meant nothing. I wish I could change the way I reacted, I didn't react at all. Our life was in a turmoil, but so was hers. If life had do-overs, that would be one of mine.

THROUGH THE YEARS

Linda

Two years had passed since the accident. I was sitting outside on the front porch on a warm autumn afternoon, thankful for all that we had. I decided to call Mercy, the woman who had prayed with us and befriended us, during Scott's time in the hospital. I saved her note with her phone number in my wallet all this time. I hadn't spoken to her since Scott had left in December 2004, but still did not feel awkward about calling. It was with that phone call that she told me the story of why she was there that night.

Mercy had worked at the hospital for years. She was a CNA (Certified Nurse's Assistant), working every night on the seventh floor in the oncology unit. The night Scott was rushed to the emergency room was no different. She was where she always was. Around 3:00 a.m. that evening, her supervisor told her to go down to the fourth floor to the trauma unit and see if she might be able to help out there because there wasn't much to do on her floor. Things were particularly quiet. That, in itself was unusual, but to transfer someone to another unit mid-shift was unheard of.

So Mercy proceeded to do as she was told. When relaying the story to me, she was sarcastically funny, stating that she did what she was told because she always did what she was told. She informed me that this was her nature, not to ask, but to do what was asked of her. This struck me as odd because that's exactly the opposite of my nature. That night, she continued, was different than most for another reason. That night, she didn't do what she was told. She went to the fourth floor and, realizing there was nothing of great urgency going on there, took it upon herself to go to the emergency room to see if there was anyone there that needed her help. As she explains it, as the elevator doors opened, she caught a glimpse of the monitors over Scott's bed, not yet knowing who was in the bed, yet knowing for sure that whoever it was, that was her purpose for being there.

As time went by, things got better. We no longer asked ourselves each night to count the improvements. Scott was back and improving more each day. Now we became the critics. We wanted our marathon runner, our weightlifter, and our wrestler back. Mike used to tell Scott all the time, "Work that arm, you need to be able to throw a baseball to your son someday. You are not left handed...use your right hand." Scott had become comfortable with using his left hand for mostly everything. Mike wouldn't have it. He pushed Scott more. Since Scott had run the marathon through the first three years of college, his intent was to run in his senior year also, but clearly, that did not happen. The following year, he was unable to run as well. Mike made a promise to Scott, so many months ago, when he was holding on and fighting to come back. He said that if Scott was unable to make that fourth marathon, that he would run it for him. This was a huge promise. Mike was creeping up on fifty, had never run more than a few miles in his life, and although a very strong and powerful guy, he did not have a runner's physique, not at all. He is a retired marine. He flew CH53-E's back in the 80's and has long told our kids, the stories of Officer Candidate School (OCS). The way he tells it, he was the slowest in the group, but in his defense, he was also the strongest. They would load him up with all the extra equipment, he was the mule, and they would begin their five-mile forced march through the woods of Quantico, Virginia. So this was a really big promise. The Boston Marathon is run every year on Patriot's Day. The first year after Scott's injury was not the time to make good on his promise. Scott still had major obstacles to overcome, before there was time for anything else. But 2006 would be the year for Mike. He started training in the summer of 2005. He started out running short distances, a mile or two, and continued on until he was ready. He ran the 2006 Boston Marathon with my son Michael; for Michael, it was his sixth time running. Kyle had been at so many marathons for so many years. The first few years he was in a stroller watching. He was not thrilled about spending another day watching. He wanted to run, but at nine years old, this was not happening. Kyle grew up with much older siblings and never seemed to understand that he was the little guy. He thought whatever my brothers do, I can do also, no need to wait ten years. The Boston Marathon had become a tradition in our family for many years. Michael started the tradition his first year in college. When Scott was old enough, the two of them ran it together as bandit runners. We would all go to watch. Our day would begin in Hopkinton. Each year was different than the one before. Being springtime in New England, you could never count on the weather. Some years, it was gym shorts and tee shirts and other years they would start the race with a hat, gloves, and running pants. Michael and Scott were in the habit of writing their names on their chests. This was so the girls at Wellesley College would scream their names as they ran by at mile 18. Any male that has run this marathon knows what to expect when jogging by the Women of Wellesley. I say jogging, not running because I've heard the pace slows down at that point, so as to take in the beautiful girls in their shorts and tank tops. If time was an issue, it wasn't at that point, at least not for my guys. In 2006, when Michael ran it with Mike, he ran ahead at mile 18, evidently sometimes the remarks, even if complimentary, were not the kind you wanted to hear in front of your father. Although the weather on those April mornings was always unpredictable, the sights and sounds remained the same year after year.

The camaraderie and the energy of the runners, as well as the wheelchair participants, was something you could feel as you walked through the common waiting for the start. For avid runners, competitive athletes, and even the spectators, there was a sense of pride, in the occasion, the event, and the country, that was emphasized only by the phenomenal rendition of the national anthem sung year after year by the same state trooper, Sgt. Dan Clark.

After many grueling hours, we made our way to meet Mike at the finish line. The crowds had dissipated at this point, but that didn't matter. We were there to meet the husband and father that had given his all to do this for his son. I was so proud of Mike that day, for the promise he had made and honored, but mostly for something I'm not sure I ever fully understood, but I felt it nonetheless. I think it was a promise between a father and his son and it mattered so much to both of them. There was a bond so strong between the two of them that even the toughest of times couldn't break it. Patriot's Day 2006 will long be remembered in our home.

April 2007, miracles really do happen. Scott, his father, his brother Jason, sister Jen, and Jen's boyfriend Josh (now husband) ran the Boston Marathon. Michael was unable to run that year. It was cold, rainy, and not the best of days. Scott had his worst time ever. The sun was going down, the streets of downtown Boston abandoned, and the staging set up for the crowds at the finish line was being disassembled. As he ran, rather crawled across the finish line, his right arm was locked (spasticity). Fortunately for Scott, this condition had diminished to the point that it only occurred during exercise. But none of this mattered, today was a triumphant day.

WALK THIS WAY

Scott

Running the marathon was a huge accomplishment for me. It was great, but I needed so much more than that. It's the little nuances that bring someone back to where they were before, the subtle things. Anyone who is familiar with the 90's sitcom *Seinfeld* may have heard of the "Summer of George" episode. In this particular episode, Elaine becomes enemies with her coworker because she criticized her way of walking. She seemed to be carrying "invisible suitcases." That was me, that was my walk. My arms were held so stiffly that it affected my legs. I had somehow gone from a wheelchair, to a walker, to walking independently, but with a bad limp, to this newer version. While my staggered stride was extremely noticeable to both myself and others, I couldn't comprehend how to gracefully walk without a dip in my hip because I grew so accustomed to not moving my arms. It wasn't until my father made the "recommendation," a term I use loosely, it was more like an executive decision, to have me walk a few laps around the downstairs of our home. The few laps turned into many more, night after night. Frustrated and aggravated, I argued that this ritual was a waste of time, turns out it wasn't. Now I can watch the "Summer of George" episode and laugh. This is the rehabilitation that many don't hear about, that others less fortunate never receive rehabilitation under duress, it was one of many.

LEARNING TO LIVE AGAIN

Scott

Anyone who has undergone a life-threatening injury and has been down the subsequent road of recovery may have heard the analogy that 'the road to recovery is a marathon not a sprint.' I can say with 100 percent certainty that this is true in so many ways.

The time to move on was now. Time to start a career, start dating, and start living again. I made a conscious decision not to discuss my injury or my last couple of years. New friends, first dates, job interviews, no one needed to know. This resolution was made rather easily but proved very difficult to actually carry out. Cleaning up my resume and signing up for Match.com were two fairly simple tasks. But I soon found out it was much easier to hide employment gaps in a resume than to hide a limp. The latter is hard to explain and at the time very hard to hide.

Common Questions

Job interviewers: I notice a gap in your resume, you were out of college a couple of years and not working, can you explain that void? What were you doing?

First dates: I notice you're limping. Why?

There was probably never any negative intent behind these questions, just harmless questions, but to me they were not harmless. I didn't want to be branded with a tag, to be thought less of. Just let me be like everyone else. I don't want to stand out.

Once I had eventually navigated the interviewing process and knew the quick answers to the common queries, I landed a job. This afforded me the opportunity to move out of my parents home into a small studio apartment a couple of towns away. My apartment was great, complete with a pool, basketball court, and nearby gym. It was only a five-minute walk to the train station, commuting to Boston and Providence. I was given the freedom of working a steady nine to five, Monday through Friday job just outside Providence. I can still recall how much it pleased me. I was doing trivial office work in a cubicle, following a routine, and like so many in corporate America, I was even given a corporate employee ID#. I had made the successful transition from having the Scarlet Letter, "TBI" over my head to just being a number. I had yearned to be treated like everyone else. My right eye needed cosmetic surgery (subsequently repaired) and my limp, which was very prevalent at the time, caused me to feel that I was being discriminated against over and over again. In looking back now, I can say that often times, that was the case, but equally as often it was probably someone making an innocent remark, but the remark along with my lack of confidence was more than I could bear. I wanted so to blend in, go unnoticed. It's funny what you wish for at different times in your life. Now years later, the last thing I want is to be like everyone else. I want to stand in front of a crowd, and be recognized for who I am and what I'm doing.

THE POWER OF LOVE

Linda

Sometimes, life plays tricks on you. I grew up as the middle daughter with two sisters in a middle-class family with two loving parents. My father was a thirty-year veteran of the Boston Police Department and my mother a stay-at-home mom like many of that generation. But unlike many, my parents were in love with each other and devoted to their children, always. Mike, on the other hand, grew up as the second oldest of six children, with an alcoholic father and a pretty rough childhood, an ex-marine, a man's man, and yet he is the sentimental soul. He has always lived by this quote. "Take a second... A second to remember this moment, this hour, this day, for this one is special, this one matters, don't let it pass you by without taking the time to remember how precious this moment is." Doesn't exactly sound like the words of a retired United States Marine. That's because life plays tricks on you. Things are not always as they seem.

DREAM ON

Scott

Dreams...We all have them and they change over the course of time. Seldom do teenagers with specific career paths end up staying the course. My dream job from a very early age was to be a police officer. My education was lining up to positively affect individuals one life at a time. Whether the effect was to create a visible presence to detract from risky behavior or help in saving lives in any number of situations that might come up. Since my injury, my dreams have changed, and while I have the utmost respect for law enforcement (with a minor degree of envy), I have changed my life's direction while not changing my personal mission.

Sometimes in life, we never quite know where we are going or how exactly we got to a particular point, but when we get there..., in moving on, we know it's right.

So needles, snakes, and heights, are all common fears anywhere in the world. Nobody enjoys getting shots (needles) and there are few individuals who would be calm when crossing paths with a snake (just ask Indiana Jones), but there is one fear that surpasses all others regardless of cultural backgrounds, the fear of public speaking. This was mine and it was real.

I was a junior in high school and running for state office in Massachusetts DECA, an association of marketing students. I'm not sure I knew exactly what I was getting into until there was no turning back. During my campaign, it was required that I address thousands of high school students and administration for this state-wide election. I lost the election but gained much more. I developed a certain swagger, a certain confidence that would prove useful years later.

It wasn't until a year or so after my injury that I approached Paula O'Connor, an employee at Becker College and a friend's mother about possibly giving a talk/informal speech to the students of my alma mater with the hopes of preventing my nightmare from becoming another's...or worse. Without any hesitation, she pointed me in the right direction for contacting the proper channels. One of the benefits of attending Becker College was that the two small campuses in Leicester and Worcester formed one pretty good size community. At Becker, you had a name, not a number. It was safe to say that everyone at Becker was familiar with my story, but now, they were going to hear it from me. And so, on April 4, 2006, I presented my first program to Becker College. This was the catalyst for my career as a motivational speaker.

I always loved to be the center of attention, but now I felt I had something meaningful to talk about. Maybe I could make others listen, so they might be spared. I knew I could make this work. My time at Expert Satellite and my outgoing in your face personality paid off. I hit the phones again, only this time it was for me. I began cold calling and emailing schools all over the Northeast; high schools, colleges, and universities. I would tell them my story, talk about my presentation and ask for a chance to speak. I knocked on doors and met with anyone who would give me the time of day. It started slowly, but little by little I felt it taking hold.

After I grew comfortable sharing my story with large audiences, I realized that making a full-time profession as a public speaker was not going to be a career obtained overnight. My brother, Michael who I could always turn to with any problem and expect positive words of encouragement was also there to give me a reality slap when my head got too big (#deflatemyego). This meant taking many part-time, per diem jobs while pursuing my long-term goal. One of the jobs I took was as a substitute teacher in a few school districts which kept me working almost full time during the school year.

During summers, I enjoyed teaching English as a second language in the United States and abroad. My first time living and working outside the U.S. was while I was teaching in Beijing for a few months in the summer of

2011. I was visited by Jay, who was bitten by the travel bug. We did some sight-seeing together on his way to Seoul, South Korea (it was a big bug that bit him).

Just as my recovery took a path all its own, so did my career, things were beginning to work out.

Now, as a public speaker, it is my hope that I am touching individuals, one audience at a time. Either by providing hope during trying times for those who have been injured or their families, or enlightening others through the verbal recreation of a portrayal of the cause and effect of irresponsible decisions through the sharing of my story. My goal has not changed. To be proud of what I do and to make those that matter most to me, proud of who I am.

The English author, Douglas Adams, whose most noteworthy professional accomplishment was when he wrote *The Hitchhiker's Guide to the Galaxy,* most accurately sums up my life when he said, *"I may not have gone where I intended to go, but I think I ended up where I needed to be."*

ON THE ROAD AGAIN

Scott

Fast forward, no longer wishing to just be a number, I began my new career.

Now I am center stage, and not only comfortable with this role, I am thoroughly enjoying it. I speak all over the country at venues both large and small. An audience of one or one thousand, from high schools, colleges, and universities to political venues sponsored by DA's offices, state-mandated programs, and rehabilitation programs. I love what I do and feel privileged for the opportunity to do it.

I caused my family some of the worst pain imaginable. Young people, people of all ages, need to think about this and the nightmares they can bring to those they love the most.

One night so many years ago, my brother Michael, sister Jen, and my younger brother Jason had the horrific job of emptying out my dorm room, loading up the family truck, and bringing everything home to a family ravaged by grief and despair. On that rainy September night, my seven-year-old baby brother was rushed to the hospital. He kissed my bloody forehead and told me he loved me. I'll never forgive myself for that and I'll never forget, but I have moved on.

IT'S GONNA BE A GOOD LIFE

Scott

"It's gonna be a good life." That was the theme song at Michael's wedding. He met the love of his life, Johnna, and married her about two years ago. I made it. I stood next to him as Best Man at his wedding. Jen married her high school sweetheart, Josh about three years ago. One of the theme songs at their wedding was "Through the Years." Jen changed some of the lyrics and had the band adapt it from the "two of us" to the "five of us." In doing so, she spent a few minutes dancing with each of her four brothers to the words of the song appropriate to their/our relationship. Sometimes, it's big moments in our lives that mark us that tend to make up the fabric of who we are. Other times, it's smaller ones. Those moments at my siblings' weddings, however small they were, they are so much a part of who I am. My accident and subsequent recovery is also a large part of who I am. For years, I tried convincing others that nothing had changed, that I was the same as before. But I'm not, I know that now, I'm stronger in some ways, weaker in others, and definitely more compassionate.

I no longer need to interject myself into conversations that I know nothing about, never knew anything about, only to prove to myself and others that I'm as good as I once was. No more. I'm better than I once was, because all of our experiences, large and small, make up the fabric of who we are.

Jen and Josh are expecting their first child in April. (I'm going to be an awesome uncle!) Our family is growing, our lives are moving forward, and I'm a part of it, a big part.

So here I am, feeling thankful, forever thankful. My life is good, damn near great! My future looks bright. What not so long ago were my hopes and dreams are now my reality. I have just signed on as an in independent contractor with Anheuser-Busch (A-B). Although I have been publicly speaking since 2006, I now have the opportunity to take my message to more audiences, to travel greater distances and to spread the word to so many more through the backing of A-B and more particularly, its Corporate Social Responsibility Program. A-B's mission "to become the best beer company in a better world" personifies the essence of my individual goals mentioned in the previous chapter, 'to be proud of what I do and make those that matter most proud of me.' At the time of my injury and throughout my recovery I learned to fully comprehend and appreciate the true meaning behind the phrase, "It takes a village." It truly did take a village, beginning with my family to bring me back. Now it is my turn to "Pay it Forward" and with A-B's power to promote, my message will be louder and clearer than ever before.

If my story can save one life or one family from the grief that mine endured, if I can stir up the emotions of one teenager enough as to have him postpone drinking until he is old enough both legally and emotionally to handle it, if I can stand on stage and espouse the need for designated friends and only one student really listens to my message, then I have made a difference. I cannot imagine a more rewarding career.

While addressing high school, college, and university students in my interactive program, *I Got Lucky!*, I discuss the consequences of poor decisions made under the influence of alcohol. I've also spoken on behalf of District Attorney's Offices, SADD (Students Against Destructive Decisions) chapters, state-wide conferences, and brain injury associations as part of the Refuse-2-Use, KEYS (Keep Every Youth Safe) and BAR (Brains at Risk) programs.

Although the name of my presentation is a tongue-in-cheek innuendo, I do realize that it is a spot on moniker. I truly did "get lucky" in that I escaped my nightmare with my life in tact and without any long-term disability. I have both the privilege and honor of serving on the Regional Board of Directors for Easter Seals of Massachusetts planning statewide events and promoting equal opportunities for people with disabilities to live, learn, work and play.

They say the harder the battle, the sweeter the victory. If that is true, I can't imagine life any sweeter than it is today.

EPILOGUE

Simply Survival or Real Recovery
Who Decides?

September 18, 2004, was a cold rainy night; in fact, hurricane winds were in the forecast. You would think the cold winds and heavy rain would keep most folks inside, but that wasn't the case, at least not for this twenty-one year old college senior.

After one too many drinks and a false sense of courage, I made what was to be the worst decision of my life. I locked my keys inside my dorm and foolishly decided to scale the rooftop to retrieve them. Seconds later, I felt myself slipping hitting the pavement below, taking the brunt of the fall to my head from three stories up.

Fast forward, at 3:00 a.m. that Saturday morning, I was pronounced brain dead.

"Brain Injury Awareness" means nothing to some and so much to others. I believe my story needs to be told for the young students, like I once was, feeling invincible, for the young men and women returning from Iraq and Afghanistan who served their country with honor, and for so many others.

I have to tell you that the twenty-one-year-old "brain dead" young man is not dead. I am thirty years old with an exciting career, and loving my life. Since my accident, I have experienced months in the hospital, numerous surgeries, and years of rehabilitation. I have met others who have endured similar injuries. I am not alone.

According to the Centers for Disease Control and Prevention, an estimated 1.7 million people sustain TBI annually in the United States. About 75 percent of the TBIs that occur each year are concussions or other forms of mild TBI. That leaves 25 percent of 1.7 million—approximately 425,000 people—with severe TBIs. Of them approximately 52,000 die, with 373,000 individuals surviving. There is very little data, if any, on those who have recovered or the extent of their recovery. Real recovery is possible. The general public needs to know this, insurance companies need to acknowledge this, and the medical professionals, who save so many lives, they especially need to know this. Those surgeons, who dedicate their lives to healing others, need to understand that maybe much more often than they know those lives they saved one night long ago in an operating room—many of them really do get to live again, not just exist!

Dr. Gerald McGillicuddy, neurosurgeon from UMass Medical Center–University Campus in Worcester, is my saving grace. On that night in September, his compassion and expertise saved my life and kept my family whole. I owe my life to him. But even he was quick to let me know that had it not been for my parents' pleas to operate, to try anything to save me, he might not have done so.

For those who have lived this nightmare or have witnessed a loved one endure this experience, for the caregivers, but even more so for the medical professionals, the doctors, nurses, rehabilitation specialists, and the first responders, please know that your work is not in vain. Please know that every day with every new medical advancement, there will be more and more like me, those who truly do beat the odds, thanks to all of you. Real recovery is possible, not just simply survival!

Many thanks to: Tobias Aigner, Sybille Fanelsa, Jens Franke,
Karen Krämer, Wim van den Bergh, Kurt Schnürpel,
Balkrishna V. Doshi, Vastu Shilpa Foundation

Contributors: Marlen Beckedahl, Anthea Dirks, Niklas Fanelsa,
Marius Helten, Nina Ismar, Julia Kaulen, Rene Kistermann,
Diana Köhler, Viola Liederwald, Seeja Lorenzen, Björn Martenson,
Benjamin Möckl, Dilara Orujzade, Rebecca Tritscher, Leonard Wertgen,
Anna Wulf, Patrick Zamojski

Photographs: Niklas Fanelsa, Marius Helten, and Björn Martenson
with the exeption of: p.2: Anna Wulf, p. 32, p.44: Nina Ismar,
p.72: Seeja Lorenzen, p.112: Viola Liederwald, p.132: Marlen Beckedahl

Colophon

Authors: Niklas Fanelsa, Marius Helten, Björn Martenson, Leonard Wertgen

Editor: RWTH Aachen University, Faculty of Architecture, Chair of Housing and Basics of Design, Univ.-Prof. ir. Wim van den Bergh

Graphic advisor: Belgrad Creative
Copy editing: Janet Hatfelt
Proofreading: Yuma Shinohara

Typeface: Lile
Paper: Munken Pure 1,3
Printer: GRASPO CZ

This publication was made possible by the generous support of:

RWTH AACHEN UNIVERSITY   FSB www.fsb.de   Freunde des Reiff e.V.

© 2015 Ruby Press Berlin
© the contributors for their texts and images

Ruby Press
Schönholzer Str. 13/14
10115 Berlin
Germany
www.ruby-press.com

Printed in Czech Republic
ISBN 978-3-944074-10-8

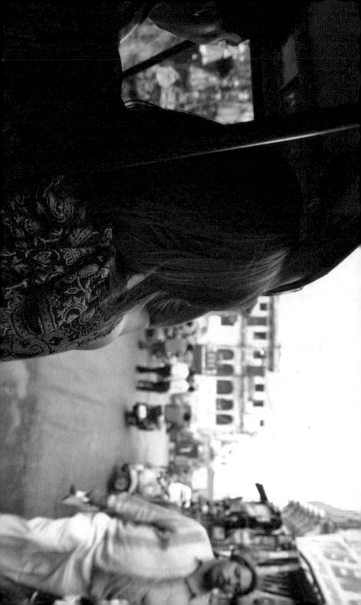